DOCTOR'S LIFE BEYOND

A true story with researches on life after death

DOCTOR'S LIFE BEYOND

A true story with researches on life after death

M.J. ZITNANSKY

Rushmore Press LLC
www.rushmorepress.com
1 888 733 9607

Copyright © 2019 by M.J. Zitnansky.

ISBN   Softcover   978-1-950818-01-3

All rights reserved. No part of this publication may be reproduced, distributed, or transmitted in any form or by any means, including photocopying, recording, or other electronic or mechanical methods, without the prior written permission of the publisher, except in the case of brief quotations embodied in critical reviews and certain other non-commercial uses permitted by copyright law.

Printed in the United States of America.

M.J. Zitnansky is also the author of the book of poems under the title *Sleepless Nights*.

The scripture references in this book are according to the Jerusalem Bible, Reader's Edition.

Darton, Longman & Todd Ltd. (1968), Doubleday & Company Inc., Garden City, New York

In loving memory of my husband.
I dedicate this book to my children Martin, Daniel, and Monica.
To my grandchildren.
To Grace, my daughter-in-law and
Martin Dykstra, my son-in-law.

—M.J. Zitnansky

My thoughts are not your thoughts, my ways not your ways—
it is Yahweh who speaks.
Yes, the heavens are as high above earth as my ways are above your ways,
my thoughts above your thoughts.

—Isaiah 55:8–9

Do not let your hearts be troubled. Trust in God still, and trust in me. There are many rooms in my Father's house; if there were not, I should have told you. I am going now to prepare a place for you, and after I have gone and prepared you a place, I shall return to take you with me; so that where I am, you will be too. You know the way to the place where I am going.

—John 14:1–4

Dying is a part of living.
We should not be afraid to die because just as
Birth is a natural process of life, death also is
Natural process of life.

To My Beloved Husband

God let you live and prosper,
Then He let you be with me.
He let you die and took you home,
But you took with you a part of me.

You love me, I know, and the love is mutual,
And this is the way it will always be.
When the Father took you home,
He did not think of the rest of me.

The rest of me is struggling to be proper.
I wish you would be with me.
The Father will call and take me home,
But only when it is time to go for me.

I have your children, their hearts are painful,
They show respect and love to me.
I love them too but they left my home,
I know that one day you will be back for me.

To know Father's plan would be helpful,
But He doesn't reveal it to you or me.
I know that He wants to bring me to His home,
And that we will be together always, you and me.*

---

* Published in the book of poems under the title *Sleepless Nights* by M.J. Zitnansky

When We Walked the Road Together

When we walked the road together,
I had you by my side,
Then Father called you home,
And I lost my joy and pride.

You left me in pain,
I was crying and alone.
I sensed the love that you send me from above,
I knew I had to get up and go.

My pain is greater than I can bear,
I know you don't want me to cry.
I know you want to be proud of me,
I know I have to get up and try.

When we knew you would be taken away from us,
We did not want to let you go,
But it is all in the Father's plan.
These were seeds already sewn.

I try to be good and do good deeds,
To see and not to live as the blind.
You came and told me "Live,"
I know that's why I was left behind.

On sleepless nights you come to me,
I know you are near.
I have to get up and write the rhymes,
That you whisper in my ear.[†]

[†] Published in the book of poems under the title *Sleepless Nights* by M.J. Zitnansky

Contents

Foreword 15
Preface 17
Acknowledgments 19
To the Reader 21
Introduction 23

How He Came to Be 41
My Reason for Doing Research into the Afterlife 55
Research into the Afterlife 67
   Life after Life: The Investigation of a Phenomenon—
      Survival of Bodily Death 69
   On Life after Death 74
   The Truth in the Light—An Investigation
      of Over 300 Near-Death Experiences 81
   Toward the Light 83
   Eternal Life: A New Vision 84
   St. Thomas Aquinas and His Work 87
   What Happens When We Die 90
   Light and Death—One Doctor's Fascinating Account
      of Near-Death Experiences 94
   The Mystery of the Mind 98
   No Man Alone: A Neurosurgeon's Life 102
   Beyond Death's Door 104

*Life at Death: A Scientific Investigation
    of the Near-Death Experience* 114

*The Cell's Design: How Chemistry Reveals
    the Creator's Artistry* 119

*The Spiritual Doorway in the Brain:
    A Neurologist's Search for the God Experience* 123

*The Language of God: A Scientist Presents
    Evidence for Belief* 125

Quantum Physics and Theology: An Unexpected Kinship 132

The Philosophical Writings of Descartes, Volume I and II 136

Republic 140

Life after Death: The Burden of Proof 143

Promise of Mercy 145

90 Minutes in Heaven: A True Story of Death and Life 148

The Young Augustine 155

*At the Hour of Death or What They Saw
    at the Hour of Death* 157

Jung on Death and Immortality 158

Into the Light 162

Heaven Is for Real 168

Why Should We Believe in Life after Death? 171
The Epilogue 179
References 193
My Message to the Reader 197

Foreword

This book is a true story with research into the afterlife. It is a lesson of courage, love, and hopes of a medical doctor who was loved by so many of his patients and who took care of his patients until his last strength. The book is based on authentic evidence of the doctor's existence given to his wife after his bodily death. It includes research of some doctors and scientists from different countries and among different religions showing the scientific evidence of the afterlife presented by the doctor's wife.

Preface

I could not imagine life without my husband. Since we got married, we were always together. I worked for him in his medical office as a secretary. We were together in the cottage on the weekends, and sometimes we also cooked together. When he got ill, I did anything I could to make him feel better. His death was a shock for me. I thought I would die too. I was not supposed to die. There was work to be done by me. After his death, I experienced signs from him showing me that he still exists. I tried to find a logical explanation of those signs at first, but there was no logical explanation. I tried to have the signs explained by clergy of different denominations, but I could not get any answers.

Finally, I was able to have the signs explained by a Catholic monk. He encouraged me in my decision to write a book about it. I wanted everybody to know that there is life after death. The urge to write the book was so strong that I could not think about anything else. I not only started to write the book; I also started to write poems that were on my mind in the middle of the night. I would write the book during the day and the poems at night. I was writing the book without the knowledge of how to write it. I did not know how to type, and I did not know how to work on the computer. In my husband's office, I only used the software for billing OHIP. The typing was done by other people. I was writing the manuscript in block letters because I did not want the typist to have difficulties with my handwriting. I talked about my book to anybody who wanted to listen. I found out that people not only wanted to listen; they also wanted to buy the book. That was a big encouragement for me. The problem was that I did not know how to write about my experiences. I rewrote my manuscript three times. I had nobody to consult with. I was on my own. The urge to write the book without the delay was very strong. I made a lot of mistakes, but I learned from them, and finally I was able to finish my manuscript. I wish I could find out who was urging me to write my book about the afterlife and who was directing me during the process. I know that God works in mysterious ways!

Acknowledgments

I would like to extend my warmest gratitude to the staff of Rushmore Press. All the staff I dealt with proved to be very pleasant people who believed in me and my work. Most of my gratitude goes to Daryl Hayes, the publication manager who encouraged me all the way.

There is no death, only transition.

To the Reader

After I did my research into the life after death, I concluded that neither science nor theology can explain the unexplainable and that God lets us have glimpses of what awaits us after we die because we will never be able to explain who God is. It is impossible to explain how God created the world and heaven and how he created us, no matter how hard we try. It is a mystery that we have to live with. We should not ridicule people who have something to tell us about the unknown territory of the afterlife. We are all desperately trying to find out if there is life after death, but we do not let people who have something to tell us talk about it.

INTRODUCTION

There is one just thing in this world: everybody has to die, and nobody knows when. Dying is a part of living. Whether you are rich or poor, famous or the least important person in society, you will have to die. We all are inevitably progressing toward death, but we are living in a society where talking about death is "taboo." There is a desire for permanence in every human heart, and therefore, I hope that after reading about scientific investigations performed by medical doctors, people will be more informed about what happens to us when we die. I hope that they will talk about death as a part of living, as natural as birth. I hope that the subject of death will no longer be taboo.

After my husband died, I felt ill. I thought I would die too. It was not until I read the book *Life after Loss* written by Dr. Raymond Moody and Dianne Archangel that I realized all my symptoms were a reaction to my husband's passing. My condition started to improve after I heard my late husband one day early in the morning. He told me in a loud voice, "Live." It was said as a command. I don't know how I heard him, if it was with my ears or just a voice in my head, but I realized that I was not supposed to die yet. I also received several signs from my late husband that I want to mention in my book. St. John speaks about miracles as "signs" (John 2:11). They are events that can help us learn about God.

The souls of the deceased are said to spend an enormous amount of time intervening in the earthly lives of loved ones. They are said to be "watching over you and helping you all the time." They never seem to tire or become bored with the everyday nitty-gritty events in the lives of their loved human beings (Osis and Haraldsson 1977, 205). Dr. Osis talks in his book about physical signs of deceased loved ones. He mentions, "Physical effects as messages from the dead (clocks stopping, pictures falling, bells ringing, and so on) were reported" (Osis and Haraldsson 1977, 12). We cannot understand this life until we learn what lies beyond it, and five of our bodily senses limit what we can understand: what we can see, hear, smell, taste, and feel.

There are people who have lost their loved ones who want to believe in life after death. They want to see their loved ones again. I have researched many trustworthy and encouraging sources about the scientific investigations into life after death. We have to remember that not everything can be seen. Let us take, for example, the atom. It can't be seen, but the entirety of life is based on it. Similarly, the soul cannot be seen, but our spiritual life is based on it. I would never believe how hard it is to write a book about things that can't be explained. What happened to me can be explained only by the research done about life after death. I wanted to know that what happened to my children and me after my husband's passing was his way of showing us that he is still with us. I wanted to know what had been previously documented about the soul.

I found out that the soul separates from the body at death. It has an energy that allows it to be in different places instantly. People who have died a clinical death reported what they saw while clinically dead. It is called a near-death experience. These people reported their experiences to their doctors, who made studies comparing multiple experiences. The studies were taken from patients from all over the world. The modern resuscitation process brought back most of the people who died a clinical death. The experiences of people from all over the world were more or less the same, with a few differences. The

INTRODUCTION

number of experiences during clinical death depends on how long the individual was clinically dead. Time here on earth is also different from eternity.

I found out that no matter how you try to explain to people what can happen after your loved one dies, people can't understand it; and instead, they try to find a logical explanation. I wanted at first to include my own and other people's experiences, which are admittedly quite startling; but after I watched the reactions of people on what I told them, I am limiting my writing to less startling and more believable experiences. I am happy that I can back up my experiences with the signs that I received after my husband's passing with scientific investigations into life after death. I know that it will be difficult for some people to believe in life after death, but I hope that they will at least try to learn about it. It is very difficult to write about what happened to me and what I have found out about this phenomenon.

In my book, I will concentrate on the books that I have read and on which I have based my research on life after death, and I will also discuss the existence of God the Designer, who gave us life here on earth and in eternity. Maybe my husband had to die so that I could write this book in a simple way for the general public and for the people that have difficulties believing in God. For some people, science and technology have become a type of God. I am trying to use science to understand post mortem existence, or in other words, an afterlife. For my research book, I have chosen several doctors who partook in scientific investigations on this phenomenon; and generally, what they found was that people who died clinically and were resuscitated back to life reported similar experiences independent of religious beliefs or country of origin. The experiences of individuals who passed away from illnesses or accidents were similar all over the world. I want people to know that one very brave medical doctor informed us that death represents a graduation from one life into another.

Public interest in post mortem existence continues to grow as more people survive death with the resuscitation techniques. The condition from which a patient can still be resuscitated back to life is called a *clinical death*. What patients saw during their clinical death is called a *near-death experience*. There is another condition that will be mentioned in my book: an *out-of-body experience*.

To be able to write about my experiences after my husband's death, I had to first get some knowledge about what happens to us when we die. Near-death experiences are an excellent way to find out. The comparison of near-death experiences of adults and children are remarkable because they have similar features. I hope that more scientists and psychologists will study this area of neuroscience to bring us, if possible, more information about the afterlife. There are still many mysteries about life itself and life after death that scientists cannot solve. I think my research into the afterlife is very important not only for myself but also for everybody else. Almost all the books that I have read were written by doctors who carried out their own research. They talked to people who died clinically and came back to life. Dead people give us signs of their existence. There is no need for us to doubt, but we are still not convinced because we cannot see what we really want to see. We still do not know how we got here; therefore, we can't know if there is life after death.

The afterlife has been on the mind of scientists just like studies surrounding the mysteries of the beginning of life. Only forty-four days after my husband's death, my granddaughter was born. The day she was born may have been a beginning of her consciousness. Does consciousness begin before birth? Does consciousness develop in the mother's womb? Apparently, a fetus still in the mother's womb is capable of tasks that humans are unaware of. At conception, a baby is a new unique human being. At eighteen days, the heart has already developed a rhythm. At six weeks, the baby begins to move, and brain waves are active. At eight weeks, the baby begins to grab and swim freely. At eleven weeks, the baby cries, feels pain, sucks its thumb, swallows, sleeps and wakes, begins to develop its sense of taste, is able to learn, reacts to light, and all its organ systems are working (Ontario State Council, Knights of Columbus).

People want to know what happens to our consciousness at the end of our lives. According to the experiences of people that were clinically dead but came back to life that I read about, it looks like we take our consciousness with us in the afterlife. The study of the human mind during the dying process started to interest doctors and scientists in the mid-1970s. Dr. Raymond Moody, an American doctor, published his book in 1975 entitled *Life after Life*. In this book, he describes experiences of patients that survived a clinical death. From Dr. Moody's findings, it is evident that the dying patient continues to have a conscious awareness of his environment after being pronounced clinically dead. Dr. Moody describes how the patients separated from their body, went through the tunnel, saw a bright light, saw their deceased relatives, saw their life in review, entered a heavenly place, and experienced a feeling of peace (Dr. Moody, *Life after Life*, pp. 11–12).

At about the same time, another psychiatrist and a medical doctor, Dr. Elizabeth Kübler-Ross, published her book *Life after Death*, in which she writes about findings similar to Dr. Moody. Other studies of near-death experiences followed with similar reports. Dr. Moody's book attracted the attention of a cardiologist Dr. Maurice Rawlings, who had also experienced similar findings with his patients whom he resuscitated back to life from a clinical death. After he read Dr. Moody's book *Life after Life*, Dr. Rawlings began wondering why Dr. Moody was describing only the good experiences of patients. Dr. Rawlings had patients who told him that after they clinically died, they went to a bad place, which they described as hell. Dr. Maurice Rawlings, a doctor of cardiology, had many opportunities in the coronary care units of several hospitals to resuscitate people who had clinically died. He found that if patients were interviewed immediately after they were resuscitated back to life, there would be as many bad experiences as good experiences reported. Dr. Maurice Rawlings has been promoted to the National Teaching Faculty of the American Heart Association in 1976. He had an opportunity to talk to doctors and nurses in many countries (Rawlings, "Introduction," p. 11). He was asked many times if those good and bad experiences of patients during clinical death might not represent hallucinations induced by the severity of the patients' various illnesses or by drugs administered throughout their illness (Rawlings, p. 76).

Dr. Rawlings writes in his book *Beyond Death's Door* about the study that was initiated in response to this problem by Dr. Karlis Osis and his associates (Osis and Haraldsson 1977). Two studies were initiated in America and one in India. "*Questionnaires were received from over one thousand doctors and nurses who were particularly exposed in their work to dying patients*" (Rawlings, p. 77). According to these studies, drug-induced hallucinations pertain to the present world and not to the visions of another world of existence. Dr. Charles Garfield, assistant professor of psychology at the University of California Medical Centre, concluded from his observations that the whole quality of life-after-death visions is entirely different from drug-induced hallucinations that patients with a great deal of pain may experience. Dr. Rawlings affirms this with his own observations:"*Drug effects, alcoholic delirium tremens, carbon dioxide narcosis and psychotic reactions deal more with objects in the present world and not with situations in the next world*" (Rawlings, p. 78).

In my reviews of other books that deal with life after death, I mention other studies that were done on this subject. Dr. Peter Fenwick explains that *hallucination* is a psychiatric term where someone experiences a sensory experience that has nothing to do with what is going on outside someone. This is very different from what occurs during near-death states (Dr. Peter Fenwick, on *Toward the Light Radio Show*, October 10, 2007). Once more for all the sceptics, Dr. Fenwick points out that the lucid clarity that occurs with a near-death experience is something that is maintained by the experience. It does not become a faint memory over time, nor does it become distorted like a hallucination. Dr. Fenwick points out the fact that the near-death experience actually occurs while one is clinically dead, not before or afterward. The clinical definition of death is when there is no pulse, no respiration, and fixed dilated pupils. Dr. Fenwick compares it to people who faint. When individuals faint, they lose consciousness very quickly. Once they come out of their unconsciousness, they are very confused, so none of these states would coincide with the near-death experience (Dr. Peter Fenwick, on *Toward the Light Radio Show*, October 10, 2007).

To all the sceptics and their argument that the near-death experiences are due to the brain malfunctioning as it nears death, I would like to recommend the book *The Mystery of the Mind* by Dr. Wilder Penfield, a neurosurgeon, which is a critical study of consciousness and the human brain. Dr. Penfield has been wondering about the relationship between the brain and mind for most of his life. Dr. Penfield shows that what people see when they die for a few minutes before they are brought back from a clinical death is not caused by the brain's imagination. He found out the true cause of those experiences. According to him, it is the soul and the mind. Dr. Penfield also said before he died that the soul has energy (Penfield, *The Mystery of the Mind*, p. 48). Another book that was very influential for me was a book by scientist and theologian John Polkinghorne. In his book *Quantum Physics and Theology: An Unexpected Kinship*, he writes that not everything can be explained by science and theology. This book taught me that I couldn't explain the unexplainable. A third very important book on the explanation of a soul was *Introduction to Saint Thomas Aquinas*. Under "*Treatise on Man*," Article I of *Summa Theologica*, he writes that the soul has a body, energy, and can move. He also writes that the soul is subsistent. Thomas Aquinas's observation that "whatever is received, is received according to the mode of the receiver" helps us to recognize why some people can't understand what they learned about. It depends on the spiritual maturity of the listener (Rohr 2009, 163).

An awesome experience is to look at the stars. They have always fascinated people. I have seen a movie about the enormous space that we call the universe. The movie made a big impact on me. Our Milky Way galaxy is only a small part of the universe. Our planet cannot even be noticed among other stars in the Milky Way. I was even more amused when I heard from the producers of the movie that new stars are emerging and that the universe is still expanding. Why should we still have doubts about immortality if there is so much prepared for us? People are suffering from neurosis. Is neurosis caused by the fear of death and the belief that our existence ends at death?

My book will tell and prove to them through scientific investigations that they will live forever. Without my husband's signs through which he let us know that he exists, this book would not be possible. He loved us so much. My husband's last words were, "I love you all, but I think that I did not show it to you enough." He showed us how much he loves us after his death. He showed us that we have a soul that never dies. This should bring a sense of comfort for people who suffer from neurosis and a fear of death. If we know that there is life after death, we should also know that God created us for a purpose. He gave us free will. Free will doesn't entitle us to destroy or change what he created.

Near-death experiences and out-of-body experiences became a subject of controversy. Researchers found out that these accounts went back decades or even centuries ago. The reason why these accounts were kept under cover might have been that people who talked about this kind of experiences were regarded as mentally ill. Books about different cultures described near-death experiences in the past. The oldest reference comes from Plato, the Greek philosopher. In his book *Republic*, written in the fourth century BC, Plato describes what happened to a soldier by the name of Er. This soldier was injured on the battlefield and proclaimed dead. He was revived from death in the funeral parlor, and he described what he had seen while he was in the state of death. He described similar happenings as Dr. Raymond Moody's patients. Plato also taught that the soul separates from the body at death. The *Tibetan Book of Dead*, which was written in AD eighth century, contains very similar findings as the ones reported by people who experienced clinical deaths to their doctors in our time. According to this book, at the time of death, the physical body is replaced by a new body that is capable of going through objects without resistance. The new body can instantly travel. The individual's senses are intensified; and again, as in the near-death experiences from our modern history, people can watch their physical body from a distance. The light will give them a feeling of peace. They will meet other spirits, and they will be judged (Rawlings, pp. 48–49). All of that is repeated in all the books that I have read about the afterlife.

The historical cases of near-death experiences have fascinated Dr. Sam Parnia, and he described them in his book *What Happens When We Die*. According to Dr. Parnia, these cases demonstrate that near-death experiences are not just a modern phenomenon. Dr. Parnia came across the first systemic and scientific study of near-death experiences.

> He talks about Albert Heim, a 19th century Swiss geologist and mountaineer who had survived a near-fatal mountaineering accident. Albert Heim collected 30 first hand accounts from other survivors of near-fatal mountaineering accidents. They all had similar experiences with a review of the person's entire past and they often heard "beautiful music."

Heim's work was published in 1892 (Parnia, p. 10). Another doctor who completed a scientific investigation of near-death experiences (NDE) was Dr. Michael Sabom, a cardiologist. In his first scientific documentation of near-death experiences, Dr. Sabom looked only at a medical investigation of this phenomenon. The title of his book is *Recollection of Death*. In 1994, he started the Atlanta study. This study was supposed to be different with regard to looking at the relationship between faith, medicine, and the near-death experience. His Atlanta study goes in three directions. He explores the findings scientifically, medically, and theologically.

People can be brought back to life with the use of CPR if they have no heartbeat, respiration, and if the brain did not lose its neurological function. In Dr. Sabom's Atlanta study, there was a patient whose brain was found to be "dead" through clinical tests, and the following happened:

> Her electro-encephalogram was silent, her brainstem response was absent, and no blood flowed through her brain during a brain operation…Even if all medical tests clarified the patient's death, the patient's life was restored. Doctors can save people from death and rescue people who have clinically died, but doctors cannot raise people from the dead. (Sabom, p. 50)

In his research, Dr. Sabom found out that no scientific explanation could be found in the near-death experience. Science does not deal with phenomena that cannot be tested.

People who have had near-death experiences can remember and describe separating from their body when close to death. What people remembered after coming back from a clinical death was very vivid. People reported feeling very peaceful and wanting to stay and not return to the physical world. If people have difficulty believing that we won't die and that our spirit, our consciousness, survives, how can people believe that Jesus was resurrected on the third day after he died? Jesus's death is documented in Jewish and Christian writings. Nobody can survive crucifixion. To make sure that Jesus was dead, his side was pierced with a lance, and immediately there came out blood and water (John 19:34–35). "This appears to be the separation of a clot and serum which we know today is strong medical evidence that Jesus was dead" (Gumbel 2003, 34–35).

Jesus was half divine and half a human being. He returned to life from a completely biological and irreversible death. When I took an Alpha course, we watched a video in which Nicky Gumbel, an Anglican preacher, mentioned that Jesus appeared on at least ten different occasions during the period of forty days to more than five hundred people after his resurrection (Gumbel 2003, session 2, "Who Is Jesus"). According to the Bible's New Testament, Jesus appeared to the disciples while doors were closed. He told them that he was not a ghost. He showed them that he had flesh and bones. He asked them to touch him. He also asked them to give him something to eat (Luke 24:42). He told them, "In a short time the world will no longer see me, but you will see me, because I live and you will live" (John 14:19).

Thomas was not with the disciples when Jesus first appeared to them. He did not want to believe that the disciples saw Jesus. When he finally saw Jesus himself, he believed in him. Jesus said to him, "You believe because you can see me. Happy are those who have not seen and yet believe" (John 20:24–29). Another mystery in the connection with a new body is the assumption of Mary, the mother of Jesus, to heaven. She was assumed into heaven with her body. From heaven, she began helping people and appearing to them. She has the power to perform miracles through her Son. Mary's assumption is a dogma that historian Miri Rubin, in her book *Mother of God: History of the Virgin Mary*, describes in detail (Rubin 2009, 56). Mary's miracles are described in different books throughout history. It is written in the Bible that the disciples saw how Jesus ascended to heaven while He was with them after His resurrection. Scientist and theologian John Polkinghorne wrote in his book *Quantum Physics and Theology: An Unexpected Kinship* that we can trust what is written in the Bible. He said that the apostles listened to

Jesus, they lived with Jesus, and they saw what he had done. If they said that Jesus ascended to heaven, we can believe it. This is another testimony about life after death.

Patients who came back from a clinical death said that our new body, after we die, would be a spiritual body. The signs that I received from my husband were not scary, not even those that I received in the middle of the night. They were given to me with love. We can live on this earth seventy or eighty years if we are lucky and remain strong, but our next life is forever. After we die, we will be judged on love. Love is the most important law for eternity. God is the Maker of heaven and earth. He made human beings, who are all unique and special. Human bodies and their functions are so complex. Animal species are all so different. For example, there are three hundred thousand species of beetles and weevils alone (Gumbel, *The Heart of Revival*, 1997). Some people started to talk about "the intelligence design" in comparison to the theory of evolution. One way of seeing the greatness of God is to look at the stars. "Our sun is one of 100,000 million stars in our galaxy (the Milky Way). Our galaxy is one of over 100,000 million galaxies" (Gumbel, *The Heart of Revival*, 1997, p. 32). My husband liked to watch the stars at night while at the cottage. On one such occasion, he woke me up in the middle of the night because he wanted me to watch the Northern Lights with him. It was truly incredible to see them move across the sky. I wish everyone could have the opportunity to be part of this wonderful experience. Just as all the galaxies and stars are God's creation, we too are his creation. God gave us free will, but we should not think that we could share in God's plans or even change them.

After I started getting signs from my husband, I did not know what it meant. The idea to write about it formed in my mind. I needed an explanation, which I received from a monk in a Catholic church. He told me that love never dies. He said that the souls of our departed loved ones might be allowed to let us know that they exist. The doctor who examined my eyes because of pain did not find anything wrong with them. He asked me what I was doing. I told him that I was writing a book. He wanted to know more about this project. He wanted to know what I was writing about. I was hesitant in revealing more, but he insisted. I told him what happened to me and that I wanted to write about it. He said that I had to write the book. A Catholic priest to whom I also told about my book and complained how difficult it is to explain the unexplainable and how much time it takes told me to continue with my research. If I did not listen to the directions of those people and had just given up, this book would have never been completed. I had nobody to consult with. As we know, God works in mysterious ways. He will help us if we let him. We all have to go through a painful journey and learn a lot from life before we can do something substantial and good.

Nicky Gumbel wrote in his book *The Heart of Revival* about Paul the apostle. After his dramatic conversion, Paul spent fourteen years in preparation before he began his effective public ministry. Paul talks about it in the Bible in Galatians 2:1. Near-death experiences have attracted professionals from religious studies, sociology, medicine, psychiatry, and psychology. Scientists would like to explain near-death experiences, but they can't because these experiences are out of this world. They are not hallucinations, and the brain does not cause them. Near-death experiences need more discussions between religion and science. The mind or consciousness and the brain, according to my research, appear to be two separate entities. Many people will believe in scientific explanations, but neither science nor religion explains everything. We should treasure whichever glimpse of eternity we can experience. People who died clinically tell us that the life we are living is not all there is. There is an eternity. The signs that my husband gave me represent a victory of life over death. To recover from grief is hard work. My husband helped me in my grieving process by letting me know that he exists, but it was hard for me to understand it. After I started my research on near-death experiences, I began to understand.

My husband was a man of integrity. When my husband was dying, he told me that he wanted a small funeral. The hospital visits were limited to family members only. My husband died on Tuesday, July 31, 2007. His date of death was not put in the newspaper and was kept a secret. I wanted to fulfill my husband's wishes, so only seven patients were phoned to be informed that my husband had passed away. They were our friends. I booked only a small room in the funeral home for our family and our extended family members to see my husband for the last time. On the day of the viewing, we were told at the funeral home that my husband was put in the chapel because too many big flower arrangements had arrived, and the funeral home management thought that many people would come. At the chapel, my husband was surrounded by flowers, which were also on both sides of the walls and in the back of the chapel. He lay in a beautiful coffin, had a cross in his hands and his stethoscope at his right side. He had a little flower arrangement from me beside his head inside his coffin with the inscription "I Love You." My husband looked dignified with a smile on his face.

Besides his family members, a lot of people came to say goodbye to their doctor and friend. I could not figure out how all these people found out about the viewing because we only told a few people about it. My daughter did not allow even her husband's friends who were acquainted with my husband to come to the funeral home to keep her father's wish. The chapel was full, and the people could not stay long, so they had to get up and make space for those who had just arrived. It was overwhelming. I got a lot of hugs and received a lot of praise about my husband. Many people cried. The same thing happened on Friday at his funeral. Many people came to say their goodbyes and a final prayer for my husband at the church. One of his patients sang *"Ave Maria"* with her beautiful soprano voice. The priest observed that my husband must have been loved a lot for so many people to come and say goodbye to him.

INTRODUCTION

I was talking to my husband in my mind, and I told him that he could not hide, that the people who loved him found him anyway. He had a beautiful legacy. Many people told me how much they loved him. He was called "the people's doctor," and his patients showed their love for him. All his life, my husband was a very humble person, a compassionate and respectful human being. He had an understanding of people's suffering. He was in his office right until the day he was taken to the hospital. I knew that he was not feeling well a few days before, and I told him that he should stay home, that I would cancel his appointments with patients. He told me, "They need me." I think that because he was always very humble, he was exalted, as it is said in the Bible: "Anyone who exalts himself will be humbled, and anyone who humbles himself will be exalted" (Matthew 23:12). Many times, it came to my mind that he is still helping other people by letting them know that he is living, that he is still with us. I think that I am his instrument to convey his message: "Not to worry, there is another life awaiting us." In the time when he was very ill, he told me that he would like to help the poor, suffering people. I did not pay too much attention to it at the time, but now I think that he suffered a lot and wanted to help others suffering because he knew how it felt.

What I am going to write about is not easy to understand. I had to do a lot of research about afterlife to be able to deal with it myself. People want science to give them explanations about near-death experiences, which science cannot provide.

It is impossible for science to take us further than scientists have done so far. Before I formally start to talk about my own experiences after my husband's passing, I would like to talk about the experiences of other people. These are signs that were reported to me after their loved ones died. A woman heard her father calling her name for four years. Another woman heard her father talk to her at the same time when he died. He came to her to tell her goodbye. Her father was in Europe while she was in Canada. A son who loved his mother very much heard his mother telling him after she died that she was allowed to talk to him, and they had a conversation. A man who asked God to see his deceased wife again saw her in his bedroom. He could not recognize her at first because she looked young, with long hair and a long dress. After he recognized her, she vanished. After that, she came to him in his dream and showed him beautiful places.

A girl saw her single mother who died in a car accident sitting on her bed. The father of the deceased single mother used to drink tea with her in the kitchen. The electric kettle started to boil in the kitchen by itself after the car accident. The mother of the same person did not want her daughter to go out the day of the car accident, but the daughter went anyway. Her daughter appeared to her in a dream after the car accident and told her that she was sorry that she did not listen. They embraced in the dream. Another person reported his father's experience in Germany. After a relative died, his father heard knocking on the door. He said, "Come in," but nobody came in. When he heard the knocking again, his father went to open the door, but nobody was behind it. The same person also reported that the shelf that was hanging on the wall with plates on it fell down on the floor, but nothing broke. The nails on which the shelf was hanging stayed intact.

Another woman reported that her friend and her friend's husband drank tea together from their own cups in the morning before her husband went to work. They drank tea together one morning as they always did. After her husband left for work, the wife went to take the cups away from the table; and when she lifted her husband's cup, the handle came off in her hand while the rest of the cup stayed on the table. She thought that the cup had broken because it was very old. The wife later found out that her husband had died that morning in a car accident. A girl had heard footsteps in the middle of the night in the bedroom where she was sleeping with her sister after the death of her grandmother. She woke up her sister, and they both listened to the footsteps. A man reported that when he was a child, he went to the washroom, which had a little window. He looked at the window and saw the face of his deceased grandmother. He started to shout. His mother sent her other son to look why he was shouting. When his brother came into the washroom, he also saw the face of his deceased grandmother and began shouting.

After her mother's death, a woman got up at 2:00 a.m. to drink a glass of water when she heard a knock on the main door. She looked at the door from the window, but nobody was behind the door. The same person found a light in the wall unit at her friend's house after her friend died. Her friend died in the hospital, and the light was not on before he died. She was the only one who had the key to the house. A man visited his brother-in-law after the death of his brother-in-law's wife. They were drinking tea in the basement when they heard footsteps in the kitchen upstairs. The man was wondering who was in the kitchen. His brother-in-law told him that it was his deceased wife. He said that she would come into the kitchen and that he had heard the footsteps before.

A man reported that he was in the basement of his house when he heard a bang on the floor upstairs, as if something had fallen down. He went up to the main floor and saw that a book had fallen out of the bookcase and gone six feet away. The bookcase happened to be on the same wall on the other side of which was his father's picture. His father died suddenly, and the man could not say goodbye to him, which troubled him a lot. A sixteen-year-old boy lost his father, whom he loved very much. He had a dream in which he saw his father lying in bed, and his head was resting on the Bible that the boy had given him as a present. His father told him, "I love you, and I will always love you." The boy thought that his father was alive. He went to his parents' bedroom, where he found only his mother. His mother told him that his father had died. He later asked for his father's time of death, and in response, his mother told him a time that was the same as that of the clock in the boy's dream. Later on, the boy found out on his birth certificate that it was also the same time when he himself was born.

A woman reported that her clock stopped when her mother died. Another woman reported this story: "The day my husband died, I heard him in the night asking me where his body was. I told him that it was in the funeral home." She did not know how she heard her husband, if it was in a dream or if she heard him with her ears. This incident woke her up. The same person reported that after her husband died, the light in front of the house flickered, and the light bulb erupted into pieces in the basement. A woman reported that she came to see her mother who lived in Europe. They were talking about the afterlife. They made a promise to each other that if one of them was to die, she would let the other one know by a sign through coffee that there is life after death. After the mother died, the daughter poured a cup of coffee out of the coffeemaker and wanted to pick up the cup. She picked up only the handle. The rest of the cup remained standing at the coffeemaker. She thought that the coffee was too hot, and therefore the handle came off. The next time she made a cup of coffee, she brought the cup she was holding to the table, but the coffee spilled on the table. Another woman reported that after her husband died, she felt lonely. She invited friends to a Christmas party. During the party, the door opened and closed by itself. Nobody was behind the door to do it.

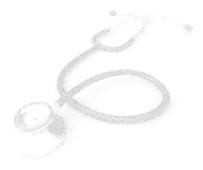

How He Came to Be

The Story of Dr. Zitnansky

$\mathcal{I}$ did not intend to write a story about my husband; I just wanted to do research on the afterlife in response to what happened after he died. I have been asked many times about my husband's life, so I decided to write a story about him.

He was born in Czechoslovakia into a family of ten children. One child died at birth, and one was only several months old when he died. The family lived in a very small house. The father was working as a rail track attendant and had a small farm with some property. My husband was the second oldest of eight remaining children; three of them were boys and five girls. My husband's name was Frantisek, but he was called Fero by his family and friends. My husband was telling me that he was sleeping on a haystack in the barn during the summertime playing his trumpet. His father used him as help in the fields whenever he was not in school. My husband always wanted to be a doctor and was a good student.

At the age of seventeen, he applied to be admitted to medical school during the communist era. During this time, you had to be selected by the communist government to be able to study. He was chosen to study medicine at the Charles University in Prague and was given a small scholarship to live on.

My husband's main interest was in internal medicine. However, the scholarship was not enough to continue his studies, so my husband had to take a break from school for one year to work in the mines. Over the course of one year, he continued his studies at the university. To help pay for his education, he unloaded coal from the wagons of the trains with a shovel and did so whenever he could. By working in the mines unloading coal and on his father's farm, he learned to appreciate people who had to work hard. He understood hardworking people, knew their hardships, and valued them. Since he came from a poor family, he was humble; this was something his patients appreciated so much. Hunger was a constant companion of my husband. Since he could not afford meat, many times he ate flour dumplings with gravy as a main meal.

At first, he rented a room at the university; but later on, when a friend got married, he let the couple have the place since they did not have any place to stay. I never understood why he did this because, after that, he had difficulties trying to find a place to live. In those days, it was not easy to find accommodations in Prague. He finally found a little room in the apartment of an old man who would play a squeaky violin several times a day. This was disrupting to my husband's studies.

Just like my husband, I also grew up in poor conditions. My father was a prosperous merchant but lost everything when the communists came to power in 1948. The only possession the communists did not take was the cottage. We had to leave Prague to live in it. The cottage was built on a hill next to the woods between two villages. Each village was forty-five minutes' walking distance from our cottage, and we didn't have a car. The cottage had no electricity or running water; all the cooking was done on a wooden stove. My parents had a small farm for food, with a goat, a pig, hens, rabbits, and geese. We grew apple trees, potatoes, strawberries, and other garden vegetables.

After the communist took our possessions in Prague, my father collapsed from a nervous breakdown. My mother did most of the work around the house, and since I was developing tuberculosis, my mother also had to take a good care of me.

HOW HE CAME TO BE

Twelve years later, my parents moved back to Prague, where both of them got jobs. My husband and I met at a dance in Prague. I immediately fell in love with him. He liked to read and talked to me about books that he had read. We both liked to go to the theatre. We always bought the cheapest tickets available, but it did not matter to us. When my husband graduated from the medical school at the Charles University in Prague in 1965, he had to do his training in the army. He was an army doctor for one year. Part of his army training was done previously during his medical studies. After my husband got back from the military services, he was working in the hospital outside Prague. He had to go to work by bus. After we got married, we were living with my parents in a one-bedroom apartment. The living room was serving as a living room for all of us and as a bedroom for me and my husband. Later on, it also became a bedroom and a playroom for our son. My husband and I were saving money for a new condominium. We had to register and put a part of the cost for it as a deposit. I have saved some money before we got married, which got handy now.

The people of Czechoslovakia had enough of the communist regime and supported the president who wanted to introduce socialism with a human face. My husband liked the idea very much. This idea did not last too long. The Soviet Union invaded Czechoslovakia and put an end to it. Many people got arrested and put in jails. The invasion was very dramatic. I can still hear in my mind the roaring of the tanks into Prague from the airport because we lived close to the airport. We could also see the tanks driving into Prague from the airport from our living-room window. People were crying and were scared. The border was closed, and nobody could go out of the country. The tanks were everywhere. I was afraid to go shopping because there was a tank in front of our apartment building. I was also worried about my husband, who had to go to work outside Prague.

The frontier was opened for a short time in 1968. My husband decided to leave Czechoslovakia and work abroad. Only people who had relatives or friends abroad could leave the country and only for a visit. They had to be invited. My uncle was corresponding with his aunt who lived in Vienna, and with her help, we were allowed to leave the country and visit her. This needed a written invitation from her. In those days, I knew how to speak and write in German. I wrote a written invitation in German in which my uncle's aunt invited us to come for a visit through my uncle because she did not have our address. We had to show this letter to the authorities. It worked, and we were allowed to visit her.

The problem was that she did not know anything about it. I had to let her know that we were coming. My uncle gave me her phone number, and I phoned her. People in neighboring countries knew about the situation in Czechoslovakia. I phoned her from the post office. I had to be very careful. First, I thanked her for inviting us and asked if she could come and pick us up from the airport. She was a very smart lady and did not ask any questions and promised to come and pick us up at the airport. I advised her in another phone call of the day and time and the flight number.

When we left Czechoslovakia, we were not allowed to take with us any documents or money. We were allowed one suitcase for all three of us. It was hard to leave Czechoslovakia. I was crying and did not want to go. We had to leave everything we owned and loved behind. My husband and I went to the Charles Bridge, which is still a meeting place for Prague citizens the day before we left. I cried and told my husband that I loved Prague too much to be able to leave it behind. My husband told me that we had to go.

When we finally came to Vienna, my uncle's aunt was waiting for us with other distant relatives at the airport. We stayed with her in her one-room apartment. We were not allowed to take any Czech or Austrian money with us. The relatives were supposed to take care of us. We had to look for work the next day. From Vienna, we wanted to go to Canada because we have heard from our friends that Canada was accepting refugees from Czechoslovakia. In Vienna, we went to the Canadian Embassy and asked if we could immigrate to Canada. They said that we could. I was glad that I knew German and some English to be able to speak for us. I asked if there would be some work that I could do at the embassy. They sent me to the American Embassy, where I got a job in the filing department.

My husband found himself a job at the Vienna newspaper. He was selling newspapers on the street every morning. It happened that the first day he was selling the newspapers on one corner of the street, he saw his sister selling newspapers on the other corner of the street. He didn't know that she and his two other sisters came to Vienna and wanted to immigrate to Canada. One week later, his brother came from Germany to visit us on his way to the US. He left Czechoslovakia for Germany with the help of Catholic nuns. The nuns helped him get to New York, where he got a job. About fourteen days later, the American Embassy offered us to go to Canada with the help of Americans that wanted to help the refugees from Czechoslovakia. We accepted the help and were taken to Canada with the airplane for which we had to pay after we could afford to do it. This was a big help for us.

When we came to Canada, the Canadian authorities already knew that we were refugees. We were put into an old hotel overnight. In the morning, we were asked where we wanted to go. We had the name and the address of a dentist in Oshawa, so we said we wanted to go to Oshawa. We were put into a hotel in Whitby, which was close to Oshawa, on October 31, 1968. There was a Halloween party going on that day. We didn't know anything about Halloween and were wondering what was going on. I phoned the dentist to Oshawa the next day, and we were invited to his house to meet him and his family. We got the welfare assistance from the Canadian government, and my husband was offered a free course to learn English, which he gladly accepted. The dentist from Oshawa and his wife helped us a lot during our one-year stay in Whitby. One of the medical doctors from Whitby got us an old house for a low price, where we stayed for one year. The doctors from Whitby and Oshawa and the priest from the local Catholic church got us old beds and blankets and clothes for our two-year-old son. Different people brought us household items for the house.

During the one-year time, the doctors from Whitby and Oshawa invited us to meet their families and friends. They also took us to Toronto, where my husband applied for the internship and the medical exams. All the people that we met tried to make us feel at home. We were poor, but it was a happy time for us as we had come to a free and prosperous country. One of the doctors who invited us to his cottage told us that we were lucky people because we didn't have to take care of any possessions, and he was right. We did not own anything, but we were happy.

One problem that we had was to take care of the rats that we had in the old house that we were living in. They lived in the basement where I had to do my laundry. I got an old washing machine, but no dryer. I had to hang the laundry on the clothesline in the basement. I was very scared of those rats that sometimes also came to the main floor. My husband and I had to chase them and kill them. After my husband passed his medical exams, he was accepted for the internship in medicine in Toronto. In Toronto, my husband had to go to different hospitals for training. We moved to Toronto and were living in an upstairs apartment with an Italian family. I found myself a job in the Toronto University Library. I did grade 12 English and was accepted to the University of Toronto. I was a part-time student because I had to keep my day job. My husband made very little money, and we needed money to live on. After his internship, my husband wanted to specialize in internal medicine, which needed more studies.

We needed to settle down, so my husband decided to become a GP for which he was qualified. We were looking for a place where we could settle down and open the medical practice. We found that place in Etobicoke near Toronto. I had to stop working in the Toronto

University Library, and I also had to stop my studies at the University of Toronto because I had to help my husband in the medical office. On top of everything, I became pregnant with our second son. We managed to save some money, which helped us to pay the rent for the office and for living in an apartment near the office. We had no furniture, only the beds, the table, and chairs that we brought from Whitby. We were a happy family in spite of the poor conditions. I distributed cards announcing the opening of my husband's practice. My husband was happier with each new patient that came to see him.

He soon became well known as a good doctor. He took his patients seriously, and they loved him for it. We finally started to make more money. My husband was paid by OHIP, which is a universal health-care plan in Ontario. When our second son was born, I took him with me to the office because we could not afford a babysitter. I had a babysitter for my older son after school. In the office, we converted our second examination room to a bedroom for the baby. He was a happy baby, and the patients liked to see him whenever I was holding him in my left arm while I was writing and answering the phone with my right hand. We were saving money to be able to buy a house because I was not allowed to do any laundry at night in the apartment house we were living in.

We were finally able to put some money down for the house near the office. My mother came from Czechoslovakia to help us with the children. I no longer needed to take our younger son to the office. I was surprised that the patients missed him. With my mother taking care of the children and the household, our lives became simpler. Our daughter was born five years after our second son. Our family was complete. We had a lot of challenges with our children, as any other parents. Both of us, my husband and I, grew up in the country, and we both loved nature. We wanted to buy a cottage property on which we could later on build a cottage. Our friends advised us to do it as soon as possible because the cottage properties were going up in price very fast. We found a property three hours' drive from Toronto.

The owner of the property gave us a mortgage. Now we had two mortgages: a mortgage for the house and the mortgage for the cottage property.

We were happy and made plans for the future. My husband cut some trees on the property and, from the logs, made a wooden dock at the lake. Someone gave us an old wooden boat, which my husband used for fishing. He loved to go fishing. He was a happy man in those days. We were sleeping in an old lodge about forty-five minutes from the property. Later on, we built a cheap cottage, which was rebuilt in 2003. We both liked to go to the cottage on the weekends even if it took us driving three hours there and three hours back. My husband got more and more patients. Some of them came from far away on the recommendation of their friends.

We had to buy a bigger house because we needed a bedroom for my mother who immigrated to Canada and was living with us. After we moved to a bigger house, we bought a dog. The dog destroyed everything he could. He made several holes in our wooden balcony and broke the glass door going from the balcony to the kitchen because he wanted to catch a squirrel. By doing that, he cut his front legs on the glass and had to have an emergency operation. We had to watch him all the time to keep him from to taking the bandages off from his legs. He wanted to bite any stranger who came to our house. We took him to obedience school, but he was not trainable. He loved us and protected us, but we could not teach him anything. Finally, we gave him to people that he liked; but after we brought him there and left, he cried and stopped eating. We had to bring him back to our home. When we came to pick him up, he was so happy and began eating dry dog food from my hand. This shows how strong the love of an animal can be. Only my husband could take him for a walk, but he did not have time to do it. Later on, we gave the dog to people who wanted to breed him. He was an expensive pure-breed sheepdog. He liked their female, but she did not like him. One day he ran away. He was chasing sheep on the farm, and the farmer shot him.

All of our three children got a university education. Two of them are teachers, and our younger son is in business. My husband needed a bigger office. We decided to buy a house where we could have a medical office and live there at the same time. Only six months after we bought the house, my husband noticed a swelling on the right side of his neck. He had ten needle biopsies, and all it showed was a puss. We were happy because we thought that he might have cancer of the lymph nodes. His doctor told him to go to any hospital and have the puss removed by way of a needle procedure. My husband decided to go to his doctor and have the procedure done. His doctor wanted to make sure that my husband's swelling was only puss. He needed to take part of the lymph nodes and send it for testing. My husband needed to stay in the hospital for this operation. When he was released from the hospital, he was working as usual. He had to wait for the results for a few days. In a few days, his doctor phoned him early in the morning and told him that it was indeed cancer.

The cancer on his neck was metastasis from a primary cancer that this doctor wanted to find. My husband had to go back to the hospital for all kinds of tests. His primary cancer was not found. The conclusion was that his primary cancer got healed but had spread fast into the lymph nodes. His doctor thought that my husband's cancer of the lymph nodes could be removed, but it was wrapped around his artery, and therefore, it could not be done. The only remaining treatment was radiation.

My husband underwent thirty-five radiation treatments, which left him with completely burned skin and loss of hair on the right side of his head. Despite the very poor prognosis of only 5 percent possibility of being able to live for three years, my husband was optimistic. He ate a special no-meat diet and ordered medication from the US, which was supposed to make him stronger and help him fight the cancer. He continued to work in his office and hoped for a cure. At the end of the radiation therapy, the swelling subsided. His hair grew back, and the skin healed. There was still some mass in his neck, but it was not wrapped around his artery anymore. The plan was to remove the remaining mass surgically.

Before the operation could be done, my husband had to have more tests. The tests revealed that the cancer had spread into his bones. In this case, the operation could not be done. My husband would not give up and took a course about healing by positive thinking. I took the course with him. Apparently, some people got cured from cancer that way. We tried to have a normal life and stayed optimistic. My husband talked to a man who cured himself from cancer with a special diet and a positive attitude. My husband tried to do the same. I saw him falling to the ground in front of the door to the restaurant where we went for lunch. I was very worried, but my husband calmed me down. He said that he tripped. He knew that there was a medical seminar offered on a ship to Alaska on palliative care, and he wanted to go there. He loved to travel. We both registered and paid for the trip. I noticed that my husband was very tired and was losing weight. I told him to stay home and take care of himself. He told me that he couldn't stay home as his patients needed him. He wanted me to believe that he would get well. He was looking forward to go on his trip to Alaska.

One day, he did not come down for breakfast. I looked for him and found him on the floor of the bathroom. He could not get up. I helped him into bed and wanted to take him to the hospital. He said that he didn't want to go to the hospital…that he wanted to die at home. My sons persuaded him to go to the emergency department that evening. We had to wait for the test results for the whole night. In the morning, we were told that he was dying, and there was no way we could help him. The cancer had already spread to his lungs, and one of them had already collapsed. He had pneumonia on top of it, to make matters worse. We were both devastated. All of the palliative-care places were full, and we could not get any accommodation for him. Finally, he was accepted to the hospital where he was on staff. The hospital had one room in the palliative care section on reserve for emergency, and he got it. All the doctors in the hospital that knew him were shocked that he was dying. They did not know he was ill. He was working the same as before he became ill. He was attending medical meetings, went to medical lectures, and was taking care of his patients even though he was dying himself.

I told my husband every day that I loved him before he died. I told him that we would be together again in heaven. He acknowledged what I said. My husband died the day after we made his funeral arrangements. I watched for a tear in his eye, which supposedly tells loved ones that the dying person loves them. I saw one, and it made me happy.

Before my husband died, we were all together by his side, and he said, "I love you all, but I think that I did not show it to you enough." A very interesting thing happened at the hospital while he was there. A beautiful, perfect rainbow appeared from one corner of his hospital window to another. We were all astonished and gazed at the rainbow until it disappeared. I have thought about that rainbow many times since then.

Fero was a humble man. When he was dying, he told me that he only wanted a small funeral. We wanted to fulfill his wish, but the news that Dr. Zitnansky has died traveled too fast without us doing anything about it. Two days after his death, we had a visitation for him in a small room in the funeral home, but he had to be put in the chapel because a lot of flower arrangements arrived, and a lot of people came to pay their last respects. A lot of people came for the Mass in our church to say their last goodbyes before his funeral. After the Mass, the funeral procession went around the area where he worked and lived and even stopped at his house before his burial.

In his medical practice, my husband had to listen to all kinds of complaints from his patients regarding their spouses. Many people wanted to get a divorce because they could not endure their spouse's conduct anymore. He would advise his patients against divorce. He wanted couples to reconcile their differences. After his death, I still had to go to his medical office. One of his patients came and told me that he saved their marriage. She also told me that my husband told her that he and I would never divorce because we loved each other so much. I was very happy to hear that. I think that love is the main law for people on this earth. We should all think about this law and live by it. It will bring us peace and prosperity. It is difficult to love people that hurt us. The main thing for us to do is to forgive them, and then we should try to find good things about them and concentrate on it. Maybe one day we will be able to find love for them in our hearts.

My husband let me know several times after his passing from this earth that he is still with us. I am writing about it in this book. I know that it will be difficult for some people to understand it, but what I'm writing about really happened. The body that we left at the cemetery is just a shell that hosted my husband's spirit. His spirit lives, and he lets us know about it. More research should be done about this phenomenon so that more people can believe in it and be confident that when we die, we really don't die. We will just be transformed into another being. This will take away the sting of death.

I would like to take away the taboo about death so that dialogues about death will not be scary for people. This way, people could be educated and prepared for the passing from this life to the next.

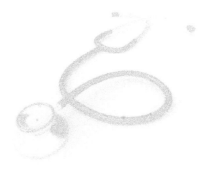

My Reason for Doing Research into the Afterlife

About six months after my husband's death, when I was still crying and felt lost, I woke up at about six o'clock in the morning by a loud command: "Live." It was spoken with authority. It sounded like my husband's voice and resembled my husband's style when he wanted something to be done urgently. No dream preceded it. I will never forget that voice. I did not know at first what it meant because I was living and trying to go ahead with my life without him. Later on, I realized that he wanted me to stop crying for him, to stop feeling sorry for myself, and to be useful. I still could not recover fully from my mourning after that command, and my mourning is still continuing, even though I feel a lot better now. This loud command is on my mind every day and encourages me to keep on living. I feel that my husband wants me to let people know about the signs that he gave me, but I also know that these signs sound unbelievable and that some people may have doubts about it. I probably would have my doubts about it too if it did not happen to me.

Since I began wondering myself what was going on, I had to do research into the afterlife. I just did not know how to do it. Since I am Roman Catholic, I wanted to know what Roman Catholic priests had to say about the signs that I received. The two Catholic priests that I talked to told me to forget about it. I was disappointed. I involved myself in a course that explained the Catholic religion.

The day the course started, there was bad weather. A snowstorm was predicted for the evening. My son told me not to go, to miss the first lesson. When I was thinking about going or not going, I felt only the urge to go. I went, and I found out that there was a substitute for the course instructor. I told him about my signs, but he did not give me any answers. At the end of the course, I was the last to leave the room. The instructor, who was a monk, called me to his desk. He apologized for not answering my questions. He said that it is not the questions but the kind of intellectual questions that I had which made it difficult to answer. He told me that if two people love each other and one of them dies, the love and the relationship still continue. He said that God sometimes allows the person who dies to let the living person know that he or she exists. This was a huge relief for me to hear. I made an appointment with him for another day, and he encouraged me to continue my research. I know now that if I had not listened to my intuition to go to the first class of this course, I would not have met this monk and would not have gotten an answer.

I continued to look for books for my research, and I found the right ones that explain that there is a soul and a mind and that there is an afterlife. It was difficult for me to introduce science into my writings. Even if some doctors that I mention in my book have done scientific investigations, I needed to investigate the science in general with regard to life after death. I found out that science couldn't explain it. John Polkinghorne is one of the scientists who, in his book *Quantum Physics and Theology: An Unexpected Kinship*, talks about science and what science can't explain. In science, the same as in theology, many things can't be explained. That taught me that I should not struggle to explain the unexplainable. I often think about the soul, but I do not know much about it.

One day I had a dream in which I saw a cupboard that I opened, and old manuscripts fell out of it. They were falling out in bunches that were connected with a rope. The manuscripts were written on a grayish-looking paper with an old-looking handwriting in black ink. I still remember the dream like it was yesterday. When I woke up, the name of St. Thomas Aquinas was on my mind, but I did not know anything about him. I could not forget about the dream and about St. Thomas Aquinas, so I started to discover who this saint was. I found out that he was a Dominican priest. He is best known for *Summa Theologica*. Fifty years after his death, Pope John XXII pronounced Thomas Aquinas a saint (McBrien 2001, 42).

I wanted to read *Summa Theologica*, but it has many volumes that I was not able to find. Instead, I got an Aquinas reader and an introduction to St. Thomas Aquinas from the library. I found in "*Treatise on Man*" article I an explanation for the soul. St. Thomas Aquinas writes, "It would seem that the soul is a body...for the soul is the mover of the body" (Aquinas and Hutchins 1952, 378). After I read this, I knew that the soul of my husband could do what it did. God has His ways to let us know what we need to know and what we should do; we just have to learn how to listen to him. If God had not put the name of St. Thomas Aquinas in my mind, I would never have known where to get the information about the soul. This information was very important in my book and for me. I want to mention now why I had to do the research into the afterlife and why I had to write the book. What happened to me after my husband died may seem unbelievable to some people, but it all happened; I did not make up any of it. My husband definitely wants me to know that there is life after death. So here are some of the signs that he gave me.

Switching of the Light, Banging on the Floor, Turning of the Doorknob

During Labor Day weekend, my daughter, her husband, my younger son and I went to the cottage. On Saturday, we went into town and rented a movie that we wanted to watch in the evening.

In the afternoon, my son and my daughter's husband went fishing. My daughter suggested that she and I should go for a walk to look for her husband and brother in the place where they went fishing. I said that I would go with her, but I wanted to go to the washroom first. Upon leaving the washroom, I went to switch off the light, but it had switched off itself. At first, I thought that it was the bulb. I tried the other switch that had a light and the heat lamp. It also did not work. I thought that it might be a power failure. To make sure, I tried the lights in the bedrooms. The lights were working. I thought that it must be a breaker. My daughter was calling me to go for a walk, so I thought that I would reset the breaker upon my return. Before I left the cottage, I tried the lights in the bathroom again. There were three switches on one panel: one for the light, one for another light and heat lamp, and one for the fan. None of them worked. I went for the walk and forgot about the light. When I came back from the walk with my daughter, I went to the washroom again. Upon leaving the washroom, I realized that the light was fine. My daughter's husband and my son were still out fishing. My daughter did not use the washroom before me, and nobody else was in the cottage before we came back. Nobody flipped the breaker. I thought that it was very strange.

In the middle of the movie which we were watching downstairs in the evening, my son asked me if I had heard a bang on the floor upstairs. I said that I did not, but I went upstairs to see what was going on. I did not see anything that could have possibly fallen on the floor. After the movie, we all went into our room to sleep. My daughter and her husband were sleeping downstairs, my son was sleeping in the master bedroom upstairs, and I was sleeping in my little bedroom upstairs. After we all were in our rooms trying to fall asleep, I heard the doorknob turning at the door to my room four times. At that time, I realized that all these events were three signs from my husband. After I realized that my husband was with us, I fell asleep immediately. It did not make me scared but happy. I know that our departed loved ones can calm us down. After my husband died, I had to go to his office to take care of various tasks. I had a lot of financial problems. I had to empty the building where my husband had his office, and I had to take care of his patients. One night I could not sleep, and I had to get up early in the morning. I was thinking about everything that I would have to do the next day, and I was talking to my husband in my mind and asked him for help. After that, I felt calm and fell asleep.

Footsteps on the Balcony at the Cottage

Two weeks after Labor Day, I went to the cottage for the weekend with my younger son and with his two relatives. We all went to my cottage first; then my son went to his cottage with his relatives later on. Before my son left, he turned on the lights on the balcony. I went to bed at about 11:00 p.m. I woke up in the middle of the night by the sound of my doorknob turning. I turned on the light, and I heard a sound behind the door like someone was there. I opened the door, but nobody was behind the door. The sound is difficult to describe. It was not loud. It was light, and I was not scared to open the door. I went back to my bed and was trying to fall asleep again. I switched off the light. While I was trying to fall asleep, I heard footsteps on the balcony behind my bedroom window. At first, I did not know what to think about it. It could be a person, but the footsteps were very regular. I listened to it for some time, but the sound was always the same. I knew by then that a person did not do it. To make sure that I was not dreaming, I sat up on my bed. The sound was going on and on. I was tired from sitting up in my bed. After I realized that the sound from the balcony was from my husband to let me know he was with me, I fell back in my bed and fell asleep immediately. This incident was not scary at all.

The Rosary

What happened to my husband's rosary is the most unbelievable thing that has happened to me since his passing. My husband hung a white plastic rosary on the rear-view mirror of his leased car, which had been hanging there for about two years. Nothing ever happened to it. It never fell down as it was not slippery. The beads were all plastic, connected by a rope. It was placed around the mirror with a loop at the post on the mirror through which my husband put the end with the cross. The cross was pulled down tightly to make the rosary secure. It would have to be dismantled to take it down. After my husband died, I still had to go to his office. There was a lot of work to be done. Each time I drove my husband's car to the office, I would touch the cross hanging down from the rosary and hold it in my hand for a little while. It gave me strength to continue my work.

When the lease of the car finally ended, the leasing company sent a person over to examine the car first and see if it was in a good condition. One day before the representative from the leasing company came, I had the car washed, and I removed all my husband's belongings from the car. The only things that were left inside it were two new rubber mats and the rosary. I left the black rubber mats in the car because I did not want the black carpet of the car to get dirty. The rosary was left on the mirror because I still wanted to use the car and hold the cross of the rosary. I thought I would take it off when I went to return the car to the leasing company. When the representative came, I gave him the key from the car. He then inspected the car, found everything in good condition, and gave me back the key.

The next day, I removed the new rubber mats from the car because I did not want to forget them when I finally went to return the car, and I noticed that the rosary was no longer there. I became alarmed because I did not remember removing it. I phoned the man from the leasing company who inspected the car and asked him if

MY REASON FOR DOING RESEARCH INTO THE AFTERLIFE

he had removed the rosary from the car. He told me that he never took anything away from the cars he inspected. I went back to the car and checked if the rosary had fallen down while he was checking the car, but I did not find it anywhere. I phoned my eldest son and told him about it. He said that maybe I took the rosary and put it somewhere in the house and forgot about it. He advised me to check the house. I checked the whole house and could not find the rosary anywhere. I checked the car again. I checked the house again, but no rosary.

The next day was Friday. I arranged with my eldest son that we would buy pizza for dinner, rent a movie, and watch it at his house. I drove over with my husband's car to my son's house. My son asked me if he could drive his father's car for the last time because on Saturday, I was supposed to go with my younger son to finally return the car. I gave my son the key for the car because I was the only one who still had a key. We rented the movie, we bought the pizza, and then went to my son's house. After dinner and the movie, my son walked me to my husband's car so I could drive home. I told him that I could not find the rosary, which was unfortunate since I wanted to keep it as a memento of my late husband and eventually put it in my next car.

My son knew that the next day I had to return the car. We kissed each other, and I was ready to go home. I opened the door of the car, and the rosary was in the corner of the carpet mat. It was intact, not scattered all over the ground. I could not believe what I saw. How did the rosary get back into the car? Where was the rosary for two days? How did the rosary get off the mirror? Everything happened exactly the way I'm telling it. None of this story is made up. The rosary was an object that disappeared from the car. It must have been handled. It must have been taken off the mirror inside the car. It must have been somewhere for two days and brought back inside the car and put on the corner of the mat that was on top of the car carpet. I was the only person who had the key for the car.

Switching on the Lights in the Sunroom

After my husband died, I found several small maple trees growing in the backyard among the raspberry bushes. I did not want them to grow big, and I asked my sons to cut them down. My sons came over on a late summer Sunday. My younger son came with his wife, and my daughter also came to visit me. After dinner, my sons and I went into the backyard to cut those maple trees. It was early evening. The sun had gone down, but there was still enough light outside. My younger son inquired as to why I had the light on in the sunroom. He said that I was wasting electricity, to which I replied that I had not turned the light on. I went into the house, and I asked my daughter and my daughter-in-law if any of them turned the lights on in the sunroom. They both said they did not, and I switched off the lights. There were six lights on one switch. After everybody left, I wanted to discard some papers into the recycling container that was in the room next to the sunroom. The six lights were on again. I had to switch them off again. This made me wonder why this had happened. The next day, I looked up the phone numbers of some electrical companies and asked the electricians if it was possible for the lights to come on by themselves. All of them told me that it couldn't be done. I realized that my husband wanted to let all of us know that he was with us. The lights never turned on by themselves after that day.

The Bible

When I was reading Dr. Maurice Rawlings's book *Beyond Death's Door*, I wanted to look up Luke 16 in the Bible where Luke talks about the rich man and Lazarus. The rich man had a good life, and Lazarus ate the scraps that fell from the rich man's table. Both of the men died. Lazarus went to heaven while the rich man went to hell. Lazarus was comforted in heaven while the rich man was in agony.

He asked Abraham for help. Abraham told him that there is a great gulf to stop anyone crossing from one side to the other. The rich man wanted Abraham to send Lazarus to warn his five brothers so that they do not come to this place of torment too. Abraham said that they had Moses and the prophets to listen to. The rich man said that if someone came to them from the dead, they would repent. Then Abraham said to him, "If they will not listen either to Moses or to the prophets, they will not be convinced even is someone should rise from the dead" (Luke 16:19–31).

Dr. Rawlings recommends in his book that we read Luke 16. I wanted to do it, so I took a Bible from the bookcase. It was a new Bible that nobody had used before. I put the Bible on the table and flipped it open. The Bible opened at Luke 16:19–31:the rich man and Lazarus. I could not believe it. I started crying and phoned my friend. I didn't know what to think about it. I told this story to a doctor who had known my husband well. I asked him if he thought that it was a coincidence. He said, "No, it was your husband. He wants you to know that he is with you."

There were other occasions where the Bible had helped me out. One day when I was baking late in the evening, I thought that it would be good to put into my book the parable of the mustard seed, but I did not know the author's name or how to find it. I had a thought that I should try it right then. I had the Bible on my table in those days, so I tried to find it. I found it on the third try in Mark 4:30–32. Another day, I wanted to find what was written about Jesus's appearance to the disciples after his resurrection in the Bible. I knew that he appeared to them, told them how to get a lot of fish, cooked a meal for them, and ate with them. I did not know who wrote about it or how to find it. I found it the same way in the third opening of the Bible in John 21:1–14:the appearance on the shore of Tiberias. Lake Tiberias is also called the Lake of Galilee. I also found the Ten Commandments in a similar way in the Bible. The Ten Commandments are in Deuteronomy 5:6–21.

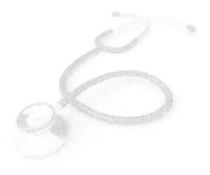

Research into the Afterlife

Life after Life: The Investigation of a Phenomenon—Survival of Bodily Death

Dr. Raymond Moody Jr.

*D*r. Raymond Moody was one of the first medical doctors to write a book about near-death experiences. He had published his book *Life after Life* before Dr. Elisabeth Kübler-Ross published her book *On Life after Death*. Dr. Raymond Moody Jr. and Dr. Elisabeth Kübler-Ross were the first doctors who investigated the life-after-death phenomenon. Other doctors followed. It is the conscious awareness of the patient's environment after being pronounced clinically dead that got Dr. Moody's attention. The patients reported floating out of their physical bodies, associated with a great sense of peace and wholeness. Most of those patients also reported a presence of someone who helped them during their time of transition from this world to eternity.

Some clergy believe that people should just "believe" rather than do research into an area that is considered taboo and which should remain an issue of blind faith. People, including me, want to know rather than just believe. When I started to get messages from my late husband, I did not know what was going on. I asked some priests what it could be, and I was told to keep it to myself. I did not understand why I should keep it a secret. Later on, I met a Catholic monk who told me that the souls of departed loved ones are sometimes allowed to contact people that they love here on earth and let them know that they are living. I was told that love doesn't finish with physical death. Love goes on, and so do relationships. The monk agreed with my research. I am very happy that I did the research and that I know that there is life after death for sure. For this, I thank my husband, who let me know about it.

It is believed that death is the passage of the soul or mind into another dimension or reality. Dr. Moody wanted to give a report on the search for cases of human survival of deaths. By the time he entered medical school in 1972, he had collected a sizable number of these experiences. He gave a report to a medical society, and other public talks followed. Soon doctors began to refer to him people who had been resuscitated and who had reported unusual experiences. There is a striking similarity among the accounts of the experiences themselves, but they are not identical. The experiences are reported in a different order, and there are few or more depending on each individual person.

Dr. Moody is trying to give about fifteen separate elements that recur again and again in the mass of narratives that he has collected. He writes in his book,

> A man is dying...he begins to hear an uncomfortable noise...at the same time feels himself moving very rapidly through a long dark tunnel...He notices that he still has a *body*, but one with very different nature... He glimpses the spirits of relatives and friends who have already died...He finds himself approaching some sort of barrier or border...He finds...that the time for his death has not yet come...and does not want to return. He is overwhelmed by intense feeling of joy, love and peace... he somehow reunites with his physical body and lives. (Moody 2001, 11–12)

In my research, I found out that people have troubles describing those unearthly experiences; and because other people scoff, they stop telling other people.

Dr. Moody talks about a "model" of the common elements found in many stories. It represents an idea of what a person who is dying may experience. The experiences are not all exactly the same. The person in a spiritual body finds that other people can't hear or see him. His spiritual body is weightless and can go through objects. People reported that there was no time during their experience. Dr. Moody found out that people who experienced a spiritual body are in agreement that the spiritual body is something impossible to describe. It is agreed that the spiritual body has a form or shape. Most of the people report seeing a light and believe that it was a being. A person is shown a panoramic playback of the major events of his life. The person is experiencing warmth and love.

People described a border or limit. One person reported that beyond the mist, he could see people, and their forms were just like they are on the earth, and he could also see something that looked like buildings. All the people that had clinical death experience had to come back. Once the dying person encounters the being of light, he wants to stay. Mothers of young children felt an obligation to try to go back and to raise their children.

Some people have expressed the feeling that the love or prayers of others have in effect pulled them back from death regardless of their own wishes.

People that came back from the clinical death had difficulties to describe their spiritual bodies. People reported a spiritual body as something that was rising out of the person's body through his head.

Dr. Moody mentioned the experience of a patient that felt like he had come out of his body and went into something else. He described it as another body but another regular human body:

It's a little bit different. It was not exactly like a human body, but it wasn't any big glob of matter either. It had form to it, but no colours. And I knew I still had something you could call hands. I can't describe it. I was more fascinated with everything around me—seeing my own body there, and all—so I didn't think about the type of body I was in. And all this seemed to go so quickly. Time wasn't really an element—and yet it was. (Moody 2001, 39)

People did not report any odors or tastes while out of their physical bodies. Vision and hearing seemed heightened and more perfect than they are in physical life. It seemed like people could look everywhere.

The ability to see things anywhere was reported to Dr. Moody by a patient who said that it seemed to him at that time that if something happened anywhere in the world, he could just be there.

People that Dr. Moody had interviewed could distinguish dream and fantasy from reality. They talked about their experiences as real events. Many realized that other people would think that they were mentally unstable and remained silent on the subject. People offer advice not to stop learning because the acquisition of knowledge is a process that goes on for eternity.

In his book, Dr. Moody writes about Plato, one of the greatest thinkers. Plato writes a lot about death, the same as Dr. Moody in his book *Life after Life*. In this book, Dr. Moody also talks about the *Tibetan Book of the Dead*, a work that was compiled from the teachings of sages over many centuries in prehistoric Tibet and passed down through early generations by word of mouth. These sagas were written down in AD eighth century. The book contains a description of the various stages through which the soul goes after physical death. In the *Tibetan Book of Dead*, the soul of the dying person departs from the body. Moody describes the experience of the soul after death as being one without a solid body. It can go through whatever materials it would like with ease and can go from one spot to another instantaneously. It may meet a "pure light." It will see other beings in the same kind of body. The book talks about the feeling of "immense peace." It can also see his life review. Dr. Moody was surprised by the similarity of the accounts of this ancient manuscript and what he has heard from twentieth-century Americans.

On Life after Death

Dr. Elisabeth Kübler-Ross

In her book *On Life after Death*, Dr. Elisabeth Kübler-Ross talks about patients who knew that they were dying. She knew that talking about death in a society that is death-phobic is a taboo and inspired many near-death studies where she quoted numerous incidents of people who were clinically dead and then returned to life. She was trying to prove that the afterlife exists. In her work, she talks about life after death, which is full of love and where we can meet those who died before us. She was trying to show people that dying is a natural process, the same as being born.

There are many things that people can't understand, and the near-death experience is one of them. To better understand this phenomenon, I will, in greater detail, write about scientific experiments of other doctors, especially cardiologists, who were trying to understand and write about this unexplainable situation—when clinically dead people can see, hear, and be aware of what happens during their out-of-body experience and what happens during their near-death experience.

Dr. Elisabeth Kübler-Ross writes that some people have described watching surgeons at work during their surgery. During the clinical death, the people that died realize that they have a new healthy body. They can hear and see again. In her project with blind people, she reported that blind people could see again during their out-of-body experience.

From her book, we can learn that in eternity, time is different. Dead people can use the power of thought to go where they want to be. I know that those things are unbelievable to understand, but they do happen. People just don't talk about it. Death and experiences of this nature are taboo in our society.

Dr. Elisabeth Kübler-Ross writes that there are people who died before us who loved us. These people are awaiting us.

In her book *On Life after Death*, Dr. Elisabeth Kübler-Ross talks about dying people passing through a tunnel and, at the end of it, being embraced by light that is extremely bright. And at the same time, they encounter the greatest love one could ever imagine.

> If someone is having a near-death experience, he is allowed to see this light only for a short moment. After this he must return. But when you die, I mean really die, the connection between the cocoon and the butterfly (which could be compared with the navel cord) will be severed. After this, it is not possible to return to the earthly body. But you wouldn't want to return to it anyway, for after seeing the light nobody wants to go back…In this presence, which many people compare with Christ or God, with love or light, you will come to know that all your life on earth was nothing but a school that you had to go through. (Kübler-Ross 2008, 10–11)

Dr. Elisabeth Kübler-Ross writes, "In the light you have to look back on your entire life…At this time you know what resulted from your thoughts, words and deeds" (Kübler-Ross 2008, 11–12). She talks in her book about life here on earth as a short time out of our total existence. She wants people to start to look at their life as something they were created for. She wants people to learn to love.

Dr. Kübler-Ross used her knowledge as a psychiatrist to help her patients, but according to her, knowledge alone is not going to help anybody if you do not use your head and your heart and your soul. Dying patients taught Dr. Kübler-Ross about the stages of dying. Her patients experienced denial and anger before they could accept their condition. Before they accepted their condition, they had to go through a horrible depression. In her book, Dr. Kübler-Ross mentions that we grow if we experience losses, if we are sick or in pain and don't take it as a punishment.

When I was reading these words, I could not understand what she meant because the pain that I felt after the death of my husband was still too fresh. But now I feel quite differently about it. I know that I have grown wiser and that I understand more about suffering. I know that suffering makes us stronger. I could not understand how calmly and graciously my husband accepted the verdict of his death. He did not complain that he had to die even if his wish was to live as long as he could in order to be able to stay with his family. The suffering must have made him a stronger person.

Dr. Kübler-Ross, with her team, collected hundreds of cases concerning people who had a near-death experience from all over the world. She writes that they all knew that death does not really exist and that death is simply a shedding of the physical body.

Dr. Kübler-Ross claims that nobody is alone at the time of dying, that every human being is guided by a spirit entity, which brings me a big comfort because I am blaming myself that I did not stay in the hospital during the night when my husband was dying. I thought that he would not die yet because people were dying there for several days, even if they were in comas. My husband was sleeping a lot, and I thought that he was sleeping. Later on, after he died in the morning, I realized that he was in a coma. The fact that he died without me being at his side still brings tears to my eyes each time I think about it. When he still could talk, he told me, "When you are here, I am at peace. When you are not here, I feel lonely." I was at his side all the time during our life together. When my husband was in his coffin, he had a nice smile on his face, and that smile made me believe that he was not alone when he was dying and that he had a good death or transition.

In her book, Dr. Elisabeth Kübler-Ross hopes that we have made a transition from materialism to spirituality. I personally don't think we have made this transition yet. I have talked to ministers and priests of different denominations, and I was surprised how little those leaders of spiritualism know about life after death and how scared they were to talk about it. I was surprised at how diversified they were and how each and every one of them were pushing his own "truth." Even among those people, it was a taboo to talk about life after death. Jesus talked about life after death himself. How can the general public know about life after death if people that are supposed to educate us about it don't want to talk about it?

If Dr. Elisabeth Kübler-Ross was still alive today, she would have been surprised at how people did not expand their knowledge about afterlife since the publication of her book *On Life after Death*. She studied more than twenty thousand people who had near-death experiences and compared her findings with similar studies done all over the world and found that the findings are very similar. After all studies that were done, we still don't believe in life after death.

I know that it is difficult because before the rosary disappeared from my husband's car for two days and came back, I was the same once, but not anymore. Why do we have to first see to be able to believe? I don't know. Maybe our faith is not strong enough. All of the work done so far shows that the dying brain is not capable of producing near-death experiences. This should make us believe that there is a soul that is responsible for the near-death experiences. I hope that my book will help people to understand what happens to us when we die.

During older times, people believed in life after death, but only few people nowadays truly know that life exists after the physical body dies, and therefore, my book will help them be educated in that respect.

In her book, Dr. Kübler-Ross later talks about our second body. This is not the physical body but an ethereal body. In eternity, we have no pain and no handicaps. Some people were wondering if near-death experiences were not simply wishful thinking. Dr. Kübler-Ross writes about it in her book:

> It is very easy to evaluate whether this is a projection of wishful thinking or not. Half of our cases have been sudden, unexpected accidents or near-death experiences where people who were unable to foresee what was going to hit them, as in the case of a hit-and-run driver who amputated the legs of one of our patients. When the patient was out of his physical body, he saw his amputated legs on a highway, yet he was fully aware of having both of his legs on his ethereal, perfect, and whole body. (Kübler-Ross 2008, 48–49)

Near-death experiences occurred at a time when people had no brain activity.

In her book *On Life after Death*, Dr. Kübler-Ross talks about reasons why no one can die alone. She talks about guides or guardian angels who will wait for us and help us in the transition from life to life after death. Our loved ones who died will also wait for us. Dr. Kübler-Ross talks in her book about a child who told her after a car accident, "Everything is all right now. Mommy and Peter are already waiting for me." Dr. Kübler-Ross knew that the child's mother was killed at the scene of the accident. Shortly afterward, she received a phone call that Peter had also died. She was aware that the critically injured children had not been informed that any of their relatives had been killed (Kübler-Ross 2008, 53). This explained to Dr. Kübler-Ross that members of the family that died before can come to help the dying person.

She also talks about a man who lost his entire family in a tragic accident. This man could not live without his family and became drunk and tried to commit suicide. When he was lying on the road, a truck hit him. At that time, he observed the whole scene of the accident from a few feet above. He saw his family surrounded by a bright light. They looked happy and conveyed to him their love.

Dr. Kübler-Ross got a message from this man who wanted to share his experience with her audience. She wanted him to come. When he came, she noticed that he was a well-dressed, very sophisticated man and not a bum anymore. This man wanted to share his story with as many people as possible. He came to share the reunion with his family. He wanted people to know that our body is only a shell and that our soul will live forever.

Dr. Elisabeth Kübler-Ross, who herself had a near-death experience, describes in her book her incredible experience with the source of light. She and many of her patients describe this light to be a form of an incredibly beautiful and unforgettable life-changing experience. She said that this is called cosmic consciousness. In the presence of this light, we are surrounded by total and absolute unconditional love, understanding, and compassion. She describes the light to be "a source of pure spiritual energy and no longer physical or psychic energy…many people call it Christ or God, since he is a being of total and absolute conditional love." She writes that we must revaluate our actions and thoughts at this time so that we will understand how we have influenced others (Kübler-Ross 2008, 61–63).

Dr. Kübler-Ross believed that every human being consists of a physical, an emotional, an intellectual, and a spiritual quadrant. She believed in the power of love. Dr. Kübler-Ross also describes what she experienced after a self-induced out-of-body existence. She shared her experience at a conference where she was a speaker on transpersonal psychology in Berkeley, California. She was given a label for her experience, which was called cosmic consciousness. After her out-of-body experience, she remembered two words: Shanti Nilaya, which she later found out meant "the final home of peace." She tried very hard to teach people about life after death. She wanted people to live more spiritually, to overcome materialism and greed.

The Truth in the Light—An Investigation of Over 300 Near-Death Experiences

DR. PETER FENWICK AND ELIZABETH FENWICK

Dr. Peter Fenwick, as a neuropsychiatrist and president of the International Association for Near-Death Studies in the UK, was able to investigate more than three hundrednear-death experiences. With the help of his wife, Elisabeth Fenwick, they described some of those experiences in their book *The Truth in the Light*. They talk about approaching death experiences and about meeting dead relatives. The dead are seen in the prime of life and healed even though they may have died ill or damaged by accidents or in ripe old age.

To do any worthwhile NDE research, Dr. Fenwick and his wife had to have a specific group of people who, as much as possible, have their NDE in similar circumstances and under similar conditions. Dr. Fenwick was particularly interested in the pastoral landscapes. The landscapes have always been described as very beautiful and usually included wonderful flowers. Dr. Fenwick was also interested in whether the NDE patients reported animals. The respondents did report animals, but only very seldom, and only dogs. Dr. Fenwick wanted to know about the heavenly music and wonderful birdsongs that were reported to him. The respondents reported mainly concordant music that was strong and emotional.

Again the research done by Dr. Peter Fenwick and Elizabeth Fenwick fits the usual near-death experiences, during which a person sees his or her body, moves through the tunnel, meets a being of light, watches his or her life review, and meets family members and friends who have died. People call the being of light according to their religion, which shows us that there is life after death for everybody.

Modern people want to have everything explained by science. Science explains many things, but not eternal things. For people that need to have everything explained by science, reading *Quantum Physics and Theology: An Unexpected Kinship* by scientist and theologian John Polkinghorne would be quite beneficial.

I am grateful to my husband that he showed me that he is living and encouraged me in this way to do research into the field of life after death. Without him, this book would not have been written. I wish my book could change people's opinions about death and get rid of the taboo and fear connected with death. I hope that people will realize that we will be judged according to how we lived our lives here on earth. Some people have never heard about it. Why doesn't the church talk about it? How could a bad person come to a good place and how could a good person come to a bad place? There has to be some justice. All the books that I have read that deal with near-death experiences (NDE) and the afterlife show that the NDE is indeed evidence that there is something like a soul, which could survive physical death.

Toward the Light

Dr. Fenwick

When Dr. Peter Fenwick was interviewed on the radio show *Toward the Light* on October 10, 2007, he was appreciated for his "tremendous amount of work done over the years to validate the NDE as automatic and real. Not being some sort of hallucination or the product of a 'dying brain'...Dr. Fenwick gave very clear, concise details about how and why the NDE is real, when it occurs and how it is distinctly different from a hallucination" (*Nightingale* 2007).

Dr. Fenwick and his wife wrote a book called *The Truth in the Light*. After the publication of their book, people sent them e-mails and letters thanking them for their work. In his book, Dr. Fenwick mentions that people's clocks often stop when one crosses over—not just digital but mechanical ones as well. Bells will go off, and animals will also react. This reminds me of what happened after my husband died. Dr. Fenwick mentions that NDE occurs only when one is clinically dead.

Eternal Life: A New Vision

JOHN SHELBY SPONG

John Shelby Spong was the episcopal bishop of Newark before his retirement in 2000. He is one of America's most popular and controversial religious authors and thinkers. The study of the Fourth Gospel, which is the Gospel of John, helped John Shelby Spong understand life after death and helped him in writing his book *Eternal Life: A New Vision*. To the question which each of us asks," When I die, will I live again?" John Shelby Spong answers, "Yes." He had to study science and theology to be able to write about life after death. Despite all the work he has done and all the assistance he has received, John Shelby Spong experienced a lot of difficulties. His friend told him that no one knows anything about life after death, and no one can find out.

Spong calls the time when consciousness expanded into self-consciousness, a critical moment of life. He mentions that once self-consciousness was established, humans experienced a "rising tide of anxiety." Spong says that death is the destiny of every living thing, but only humans know that.

I was always aware of the fact that human beings are constantly fearful. John Shelby Spong confirms it in his book *Eternal Life: A New Vision*. He talks about death as a natural part of the cycle of life. Human beings are reminded all the time that their lives will end one day. This brings anxiety to people's lives. To lower the anxiety and to be able to survive, people developed religion. This is what John Shelby Spong writes about in this book. He is stressing the fact that it is only human beings that know that they will die.

John Shelby Spong thinks that religion helped people to deal with the anxiety associated with death. He is worried that religion can die. He is worried what will happen to the anxieties when religion dies.

John Shelby Spong recognized that the most important word in the origin of religion is *spirit*. The idea that there is nothing after death was threatening to human beings. Human beings always wanted to know if there is a continuation of life after death. The goal of John Shelby Spong's book is to find out. Religions talk about eternity only in connection with the standards that the believers have to meet before they could pass into a promised eternity. Spong noticed that according to the reports of people that died a clinical death and came back, nobody was treated according to their beliefs, religion, or race. People were treated according to their deeds. Spong rejects fundamentalism. He mentions that a common DNA flows through all living things. He admits that life is a mystery that we cannot explain. Spong mentions,

> Quantum physics evolved from the discovery that atoms, previously considered to be the basic building blocks of nature could be split into particles. Furthermore, these subatomic particles were observed to act in unpredictable ways. They could emit discrete bundles of light, which are quantified packages of energy that can spontaneously transform into physical waves of measurable energy. The discoveries from this new world of quantum physics heralded the modern era of nuclear science. It is now evident that such subatomic particles are prevalent within the outer space of our universe. These particles energize the interconnecting fabric of the entire cosmos. It is this knowledge that introduced us to a new awareness that

we are not now and never have been separated or alone. (Spong 2009, 152)

John Shelby Spong quotes passages from the Bible showing us how Jesus taught His disciples. Jesus taught them about himself and his relationship with his Father. He also told them that he existed before Abraham did. In John's Gospel, Jesus makes this claim to be beyond time (Spong 2009, 169). Jesus was assuring his disciples about everlasting life when he told them that he would leave them, but he would not leave them orphans. He said that in a short time, the world would no longer see him, but the disciples would see him. Spong writes about Jesus becoming one with God by mentioning John's Gospel where Philip, one of Jesus's disciples, asks Jesus to show them the Father. Jesus responds that if Philip has seen Jesus, he has seen God. Jesus also said in this Gospel that the words he speaks are not his words but God's (Spong 2009, 168).

Spong admitted that he wanted to reform the institutions of religion. He said that he wanted to make them serve the purpose for which they were created. According to his opinion, spirituality abroad today is deeper than we have ever witnessed, but the popularity of religious institutions is declining.

By reading John Shelby Spong's *Eternal Life: A New Vision*, I have learned that he believes that the earth is the doorway to heaven and that humans can be transformed into the divine. He believes that *yes*, we will live again.

St. Thomas Aquinas and His Work

I only knew the name of St. Thomas Aquinas. I had never heard anybody talk about him or mention his works. Recently, while reading the book by Richard Rohr *The Naked Now*, I came across his note in appendix 1, page 163, in which he reminds us of Thomas Aquinas's observations that "whatever is received is received according to the mode of the receiver." What happened to me was that I had a very vivid dream one night in which I saw very clearly a cupboard with a little handle, which I opened. Manuscripts fell out of the cupboard in bunches. They looked old with black-ink writing on them. I woke up wondering what relevance it had, with the name *St. Thomas Aquinas* stuck in the back of my mind. The name St. Thomas Aquinas would not leave my brain. I looked up his name in the book that I have about saints and found out that he was one of the greatest theologians that had ever been born. He was born in 1225.

Arriving in Paris in 1245, Thomas began his theology at the Dominican convent. His master there was Albert the Great. During this period, he was ordained a priest. In 1252, Thomas entered upon the teaching career to which he was to devote the rest of his life. "Thomas Aquinas…Doctor of the Church, also known as the 'Angelic Doctor' is one of the greatest and most influential theologians in the entire history of the church" (McBrien 2003, 90). Less than fifty years after his death, Pope John XXII pronounced Thomas Aquinas a saint (McBrien 2001, 92).

Thomas Aquinas is best known for his *Summa Theologica*. The writing career of Thomas Aquinas came to an end on December 6, 1273. After celebrating Mass that day, he stopped writing. His companion urged him to complete his work. He replied, "All I have written seems to me like straw compared with what I have seen and what has been revealed to me" (McBrien 2003, 91). It is believed that he had a spiritual experience while celebrating Mass. On his way to a Council of Lyon, riding on a donkey, Thomas Aquinas became seriously ill. He died on March 7, 1274.

From St. Thomas Aquinas work *Summa Theologica*, I was happy to find in "*Treatise on Man*" in article 1:

> It would seem that the soul is a body...for the soul is the mover of the body...therefore the soul is a mover moved. But every mover moved is a body, therefore the soul is a body...Since, therefore, the soul moves the body, it seems that the soul must be a body. (Aquinas and Hutchinsons 1952, 378)

To the question of whether the human soul is something subsistent, which means capable of surviving, Aquinas answers:

> It must necessarily be allowed that the principle of intellectual operation which we call the soul is a principle both incorporeal and subsistent. For it is clear that by means of the intellect man can know the natures of all corporeal things...Therefore, the intellectual principle, which we call the mind or the intellect, has an operation per se apart from the body. Now only that, which subsists can have an operation per se...We must conclude, therefore, that the human soul, which is called the intellect or the mind, is something incorporeal and subsistent. (Aquinas and Hutchinsons 1952, 379–380)

It seems clear to me now that I had to have a dream about St. Thomas Aquinas's manuscripts. Where else would I be able to find so much information about the soul that I needed for my research? In 1880, Aquinas was declared patron of all Catholic educational establishments. According to Aquinas, God reveals himself through nature, so to study nature is to study God.

Why was *Summa Theologica*, the monumental work of Saint Thomas Aquinas, not completed? He knew that we will never be able to explain who God is. He wrote, "The ultimate human knowledge of God is to know that we do not know God and that insofar as we know what God is transcending all that we understand of God" (McBrien 2003, 91).

I am glad that I could get some knowledge about the soul from St. Thomas Aquinas's *Summa Theologica*. This knowledge is very important to me. I know now how my husband's rosary could be taken out from the car and brought back in two days. According to St. Thomas Aquinas, the soul is a body. The soul can move. I know that I would never think about St. Thomas Aquinas and his work if his name had not gotten stuck in my mind. The soul of my husband could switch off the light in the bathroom, put on the lights in the sunroom, turn the doorknob of my bedroom, open the Bible for me on the page that I wanted to find, and walk on the balcony. Richard Rohr talks in his book *The Naked Now* about St. Thomas Aquinas's observation that "whatever is received is received according to the mode of the receiver," which teaches us that whatever people are hearing is received according to the maturity of the listener. This is a very important observation to know about too because not everybody will understand what I am writing about.

What Happens When We Die

Dr. Sam Parnia

In Dr. Pernia's book, I read again that when people are asked about their NDE, they mention similar circumstances like in the other books that I have read. People go through a tunnel and see a bright light at the end. Some people may not see the tunnel at all. People can understand how their mistakes hurt others. They know that they are in the place of spirits. People from all over the world talked about seeing a lot of light and experiencing a lot of love. After this experience, people have no fear of death and believe in the afterlife. People describe figures that have white robes. Again, as in other books that are written about near-death experiences, people meet all of their dead loved ones. People are told that they will not stay, and they go back to their bodies through a tunnel. "People reported to Dr. Parnia that they were in a very beautiful place. They felt very happy and peaceful. They described misty surroundings, beautiful meadow, a garden or grasslands." People reported a point that they should not pass in the form of a stream, river, or a doorway.

Dr. Sam Parnia reports a particular pattern similar to the patterns reported by other doctors that investigated NDE as well. It is difficult for people to describe the light.

> Those who did describe it typically called it a very "warm," "welcoming," and "glorious" light that didn't hurt their

eyes, but instead drew them toward it. Many also described the sensation of separating from their bodies and being able to "see" events from below while "floating" in an "out-of-body" state. This was described as being like removing a heavy garment of clothing or shedding a skin and moving away freely, leaving the old skin behind. Interestingly, people consistently described the "self" as the part that was above, rather than the body that was lying below. Throughout the experiences, people consistently described being able to think clearly and lucidly, with well-structured thought process together with clear reasoning and memory formation. (Parnia 2006, 67–68)

After reading Dr. Parnia's book about what happens after we die, I understood that NDEs prove that there is life after death and that the spirits of our loved ones can give us signs of their existence, can protect us, and can guide us if we let them. We just need to listen to them. Why don't the religious authorities believe in NDE or the signs of the spirits? Dr. Sam Parnia mentions that NDEs don't correlate directly with traditional religious views of the afterlife (Pernia 2006, 69).

The best account of the prevalence of NDEs come from a Gallup survey carried out in the US in 1982. This survey concluded that near-death experiences had occurred in approximately eight million people, or 4 percent of the population. This survey indicated that near-death experiences were far more common than most people had thought. Dr. Parnia found that events closely resembling NDEs had been described in many parts of the world in the past and in modern times.

Dr. Parnia's study was supposed to analyze what people experience when they reach the point of death. All of the people that had an NDE in his study followed the core experiences as described by Dr. Moody. In his book, Dr. Parnia talks about cells that can communicate with one another. Dr. Parnia points out that to communicate their distress, the cells will use chemicals.

According to Dr. Parnia's study, it looks like people that had NDE also had out-of-body experiences and had been transformed in a positive manner. Dr. Parnia found out that the behavior and attitude of people that had NDEs had changed significantly.

There is still a question for current understanding of consciousness and its relation to brain function, which means the relationship between the mind and the brain. How can thought processes, memory formation, and reasoning be occurring at a time when there was little or no brain function? Dr. Parnia had a paradox that he could not understand. He wanted to understand why, when a state of confusion would make sense during NDE due to the lack of nutrients to the brain, would patients experience "lucid, well-structured thought processes, together with reasoning and memory formation from that time" (Parnia 2006, 92). Dr. Parnia did not think it made sense for people to remember the NDE so clearly. He thought about the possibility that perhaps a state of consciousness was not related to the brain. Dr. Parnia came across children's near-death experiences, which was fascinating for him. The children reported very similar experiences as adults. This was a very convincing finding for him.

Dr. Parnia realized that the nature of consciousness and the mind is one of the greatest mysteries facing science. He knew that well-known philosophers such as Plato and Descartes had argued that the mind and the brain were separate entities. By studying near-death experiences, we can solve the mystery about life after death. Modern medical equipment helps us to bring people back to life from the clinical death. Science has not found any biological substance for the existence of the consciousness and the mind. We know that consciousness exists even if we don't see it.

At the end of his Southampton study, Dr. Parnia had to accept that the formation of consciousness is far from clear. Dr. Parnia found out that near-death experiences were very popular all over the world. Neuroscience is still trying to find more about consciousness.

In an editorial in the prestigious medical journal *The Lancet*, Professor French, a psychologist at the University of London, concluded, "The nature of mind-brain relationships and the possibility of life-after-death are some of the most profound issues relating to mankind's place in the universe" (Parnia 2006, 166). According to Dr. Parnia, there is a likelihood that consciousness and the brain can be present independently even for a time after death (Parnia 2006, 170).

Dr. Parnia believes that NDEs will show us a connection between the "soul" and what we consider consciousness. NDEs hold the key to solving the mystery of what happens to all of us when we die. By studying the NDEs, we will be able to answer the question regarding the existence of an afterlife.

Light and Death—One Doctor's Fascinating Account of Near-Death Experiences

Dr. Michael Sabom

Dr. Michael Sabom, a cardiologist, wrote his first book, *Recollections of Death*, as a medical investigation of near-death experiences. He later realized that he did not consider the spiritual meaning behind near-death experiences. In 1994, he launched the Atlanta study. This study was supposed to show the relationship between faith, medicine, and near-death experiences. It took him two years to find twenty-eight women and nineteen men who had near-death experiences. Their ages ranged from thirty-three to eighty-two years. People that have near-death experiences and are in a clinical death without heartbeat and respiration can be brought back to life with the help of CPR.

In Dr. Sabom's Atlanta study, the person who had the deepest near-death experience was Pam Reynolds. All of Pam's vital signs had to be stopped for an operation nicknamed "standstill" in order to be able to operate on a giant basilar artery aneurysm. A safe removal was possible only by a surgical procedure known as hypothermic cardiac arrest (Sabom 1998, 35–37).

In his book, Dr. Sabom describes the operation and Pam Reynolds's testimony of what she experienced in the operating room while she was out of her body. Being out of her body, Pam Reynolds left the operating room, and she described what she experienced:

> The feeling was like going up in an elevator real fast...It was like a tunnel but it wasn't a tunnel...I became aware of my grandmother calling me. But I didn't hear her call me with my ears...It was a clearer hearing than with my ears... at the very end there was this very little tiny pinpoint of light that kept getting bigger and bigger and bigger...I recognized a lot of people...They would not permit me to go further...I wanted to go into the light, but I also wanted to come back. I had children to be reared...then they (deceased relatives) were feeding me. They were not doing this through my mouth, like with food, but they were nourishing me with something. (Sabom 1998, 44–45)

Dr. Sabom writes that Pam's body appeared to be waking up, perhaps at a time during her near-death experience when she was being strengthened. But unfortunately Pam had a lethal cardiac rhythm. With a lot of effort from the cardiac surgical team, Pam returned from her near-death experience.

The people that report near-death experiences apparently did not completely cross over the barrier to the afterlife. People that had near-death experiences also report this in other books. By reading about these near-death experiences, I could find out that we will live in eternity after we die, but I cannot find what happens when we cross over completely because nobody has come back from there yet. By experiencing the messages and signs that my husband was able to communicate to my children and me, I could see that the spirit can come back to earth. The spirit of the deceased person can communicate to us that we will live after we die here on earth. Many people have been brought back to life in the hospitals during cardiac arrests when medical teams immediately initiated cardiopulmonary resuscitation (CPR). These teams had approximately four to six minutes to treat the arrest before irreversible brain damage and death occurred.

In his book *Light and Death*, Dr. Michael Sabom, a cardiologist, describes how he tried, along with a team, to revive a close friend and a fellow physician. After a full CPR and about fifteen electrical shocks, his friend showed no response. After one supercharged shock, the patient's normal sinus rhythm was restored. His friend told him about his near-death experience. He told Dr. Sabom that he heard his mother who died a year ago. His mother's voice told him that it was not his time to go. After that, he woke up on the respirator. In his book, Dr. Sabom talks about other people that died and were turned back. People are prevented from crossing a barrier and proceed into death.

Dr. Raymond Moody was criticized by Dr. Sabom for not using any scientific explanations and not explaining any medical details in his *Life after Life* international best seller. After that, Dr. Sabom decided to do his own study but found out that he could not use science to explain this phenomenon. Science just can't explain near-death experiences. Dr. Michael Sabom's Atlanta study, the same as Dr. Sam Parnia's Southampton study, were both scientific studies, but they could not explain near-death experiences. These experiences were very similar. People report going through the tunnel, seeing a bright light, seeing their dead relatives, seeing a review of their lives, and coming to a heavenly place. Some patients report leaving their bodies and watching the resuscitation process. Neuroscience has a problem explaining NDE. Scientists thought that the best understanding of NDEs could be achieved by studying the state of clinical death, which remains reversible for about thirty minutes.

The patients were able to remember what happened, even in the absence of brain processes. Scientists found out that consciousness can continue to exist even without the support of the vital signs of the body. In his work, Dr. Sabom mentions Dr. Wilder Penfield, who was a "renowned neurosurgeon who spent a lifetime studying the human brain." He mentions that Penfield stressed that the soul has an energy and states that Penfield expressed surprise at this new knowledge. Dr. Sabom writes, "In my research with the near-death experience, I, like Penfield, have discovered the footprints of a nonphysical 'energy at play'" (Sabom 1998, 190–191).

In his book *Recollection of Death*, which was published in 1982, Dr. Sabom suggested that the NDE may involve God. His book had touched on "a subject dear to the hearts of all Christians." (Sabom, 1998, p. 193)

Dr. Sabom mentions that scientists have avoided dealing with the nonmaterial world. He believes that NDE is indeed a spiritual experience because decades of research have failed to show physical explanation. In his book *Light and Death*, he believes that the near-death experience is a spiritual encounter. The experiences are real, not imaginary or the product of a hallucination. According to Dr. Sabom, NDE "is an experience that occurs as the soul separates from the body in the death process" (Sabom 1998, 204).

The Mystery of the Mind

WILDER PENFIELD, OM, LITT.B, MD, FRS

*D*r. Wilder Penfield was a neurosurgeon. He wanted to find the nature of the mind in relationship to the brain. He believed that "the mind must be viewed as a basic element in itself. One might call it a medium, an essence, a soma. That is to say, it has a continuing existence" (Penfield, 1975, "Foreword," p. xxi–xxii). This happens to be one of the features where Dr. Penfield agreed with Descartes. For Dr. Penfield, the mind was a mystery. In preparation for his book *The Mystery of the Mind*, Dr. Penfield asked three of his friends to join him in the publication: William Feindel, a neurosurgeon; Charles Hendel, a philosopher; and Sir Charles Symonds, a neurologist.

In his search for the truth, Dr. Penfield found that there is in the brain an amazing automatic sensory and motor computer that utilizes the conditioned reflexes, and there is a higher brain mechanism that is most closely related to that activity that men have long referred to as consciousness, or the mind, or the spirit. (Penfield 1975, "Preface," p. xiii)

Dr. Charles W. Hendel, Litt.B, PhD, a philosopher, said after reading Dr. Penfield's manuscript that it was an inspiration and gave him hope in his own faith. He agreed that the evidence showed how the mind "is a very distinctive reality." For Dr. Hendel, reading Dr. Penfield's manuscript was a thrilling story telling how Dr. Wilder Penfield found out things about the cerebral cortex and the mechanisms of the higher brain stem that turned into a vital hypothesis (Penfield 1975, "Foreword," p. xvii).

Another of Dr. Penfield's friends, Dr. Sir Charles Sherrington, noted, "Mind, meaning of that thought, memory, feelings, reasoning, and so on, is difficult to bring into a class of physical things" (Penfield 1975, "Introduction," p. xxv). According to Dr. Sherrington, either brain action explains the mind, or there are two elements to deal with.

For Dr. Penfield, the brain is an "automatic coordinator." He states, "Mind comes into action and goes out of action with the highest brain-mechanism, it is true. But the mind has energy; the form of that energy is different from that of neuronal potentials that travel the axon pathways. There I must leave it" (Penfield 1975, 48).

Axone (or *axon*, according to the *Living Webster Encyclopaedic Dictionary*) is "a long, single nerve cell process, which carries transmitted nerve impulses away from the body or the cell" (Pei 1971). This energy seems to be a nonphysical energy.

In his recapitulation, Dr. Penfield writes:

> Mind, brain, and body make the man, and the man is capable of so much...Certainly, mind and brain carry on their functions normally as a unit...The function of this gray matter...is to carry out the neuronal action that corresponds with the action of the mind...The function of the gray matter...is to coordinate sensory-motor activity previously programmed by the mind. (Penfield 1975, 62–64)

What Dr. Penfield calls the mind and what it does is described in this manner by him:

> The mind is aware of what is going on. The mind reasons and makes new decisions. It understands. It acts as though endowed with an energy of its own. It can make decisions

and put them into effect by calling upon various brain mechanisms. It does this by activating Neuro-mechanisms. This, it seems, could only be brought about by expenditure of energy. (Penfield 1975, 75–76)

All of his adult life, Dr. Penfield was trying to solve the mystery of the mind. He found it quite absurd to expect the highest brain mechanism to carry out what the mind does and thus perform all the functions of the mind. He expressed his opinion about the mind and the highest brain mechanism in his book *The Mystery of the Mind*:

If there are two elements, then energy must be available in two different forms...and yet the mind seems to act independently of the brain in the same sense that a programmer acts independently of his computer, however much he may depend upon the action of that computer for certain purposes. (Penfield 1975, 79–80)

Dr. Penfield felt pressure to choose the proposition that our being is to be explained on the basis of two fundamental elements: the brain and the mind. According to Dr. Penfield, the highest brain mechanism is the "mind's executive." Somehow the executive accepts direction from the mind and passes it on to various mechanisms in the brain. Dr. Penfield believes that if the active mind of a man does communicate with other active minds, it can do so only by the transfer of energy from mind to mind directly. Dr. Penfield writes that this suggests that energy passes from spirit to spirit (Penfield 1975, 85–90).

It was already mentioned before in this book that shortly before his death, Dr. Penfield expressed his surprise at discovering that the mind, spirit, or soul of a person have energy. This, in some ways, explains that the messages or signs my family and I received after my husband's death was my husband's spirit communicating with our spirits, letting us know he exists. Sometimes I also feel being guided in my decisions, which I can't explain. This may as well be communicated between my husband's and my own spirit. Dr. Penfield concludes that it is easier to rationalize man's being on the basis of two elements than on the basis of one. He believed that the final scientific conclusion about the nature of energy responsible for the action of the mind would be discovered.

Dr. Penfield is remembered for discovering that the mind has energy. He mentioned that people take "mind" and "the spirit of man" to be the same. He believed that our being is to be explained on the basis of two elements: the brain and the mind. Dr. Penfield was brought up in a Christian family, and he had always believed that there was work for him to do in the world. We all have to thank him for what he has done.

No Man Alone: A Neurosurgeon's Life

Dr. Wilder Penfield

No Man Alone—what an encouraging title for Dr. Wilder Penfield's book. This American-born doctor, who became a Canadian and lived in Canada until his death, left us an incredible legacy. He told us not to worry, that we would get help in our transition. Dr. Wilder Penfield was a brain surgeon. He felt that he was supposed to leave something very important here on earth, and he did. He found out that we have a soul and mind and that they are driven by energy (Wilder Penfield, *Mystery of the Mind*, pp. 75–76). All his life, he suspected this. He was sure about the soul and the mind, but it was only weeks before his death when he found that the soul was driven by energy.

He himself was surprised that his suspicion was true. Too bad that he did not live longer to explain his findings to us. Maybe it was meant for us to do some searching ourselves too (Wilder Penfield, *Mystery of the Mind*, p. 48).

As a brain surgeon, he operated on many brains, and he could see that the brain is not capable of the usual functions during clinical death. Only with the resuscitation of the lungs, the heart, and the brain is the human body able to resume its functions. He helped us to solve the puzzle on how people can see during clinical deaths. He certainly helped me to solve my puzzle by finding that the soul of a person has energy. Dr. Penfield believed that each of us would get someone to guide us at the transition from this world to the next. He knew it because he talked to people who had died and come back. I know that it is very difficult to understand all that, but we have to try. We have to search. God gave us his Son, who taught us about his Father and left written laws and guidance. We all should take a few minutes from our lives and learn that this life is not all that exists.

In his book *No Man Alone*, Dr. Penfield writes:

> No man alone—these words have been repeated so often in the pages of this book! But one discovers that they have taken on a deeper meaning. Workers have need of the genius and the criticism of other workers, of course. But beyond that, they should come in time to read the design and the purpose of the Creator of our universe, and seek to know His will. (*No Man Alone*, p. 344)

Dr. Wilder Penfield was born in the Spokane, Washington. Later in his life, he moved his family to London, New York, Spain, Germany, and finally to Montreal, Canada. He is considered to be a Canadian. He served as a neurosurgeon at Montreal General Hospital in Canada and was acting as a professor of neurology and neurosurgery at McGill University from 1933 to 1960. He published numerous books on neurology, neurosurgery, and epilepsy. He died on April 5, 1976.

Beyond Death's Door

DR. MAURICE RAWLINGS

    Dr. Rawlings, a cardiologist, wrote this book after a frightening experience with a patient in his office. He describes what happened to one of his patients during a "stress test" performed to evaluate complaints of chest pains. The patient's heart had stopped in the middle of the stress test. It was late afternoon, and Dr. Rawlings was the only doctor in the clinic with the nurses. The patient had cardiac arrest and collapsed right in his office. Dr. Rawlings and the nurses started to work on resuscitating the patient immediately, but the heart would not maintain its own beat. Dr. Rawlings started external heart massage as soon as he could no longer hear a heartbeat and could not feel a pulse. He had to insert a pacemaker wire into the large vein beneath the collarbone that leads directly to the heart. The patient had a complete heart blockage. He was constantly between death and coming back to life. Each time the patient regained his heartbeat and respiration, he screamed, "I am in hell!" Then he told the doctor, "Don't stop!" The patient appeared to be very scared when he told Dr. Rawlings that he was in hell and asked Dr. Rawlings to pray for him. Dr. Rawlings did not usually pray, but he asked the patient to repeat the words after him.

    The patient asked Lord Jesus to keep him out of hell and forgive him his sins. He said that he would turn his life over to him. If he died, he wanted to go to heaven. If he lived, he promised to be on the hook forever. The patient's condition finally stabilized, and he was transported to a hospital. Before this incident, death to Dr. Rawlings was the extinction of the person. After the incident in his office, he realized that death should be considered something different from extinction. He started to read the Bible. A couple of days later, Dr. Rawlings approached the patient with a pad and pencil for an interview. He asked him what he actually saw in hell. The patient said that he did not recall any hell. He could not recall any of the unpleasant events! He reported that he remembered only having had an out-of-body experience and meeting both his mother and his stepmother during his death episodes. He also saw other relatives who had died before. He was in a place that was illuminated by a huge beam of light. He saw his mother for the first time. She died when he was fifteen months old. His father had soon remarried. This man had never even seen a picture of his real mother. He picked her picture out of several others later on when his mother's sister showed it to him. His mother was still twenty-one years old when he saw her, the age when she died (Rawlings 1978, 20–22).

This case explains why there are only good experiences reported by patients. When patient interviews are delayed, bad experiences are rejected from the memory by the time of the interview. Dr. Rawlings later on made sure to have interviews with the patients immediately after their resuscitation from clinical deaths. He found afterward that not all experiences are good. The reports that Dr. Rawlings collected are similar in many other reports. Dr. Rawlings writes that people in clinical death hear the doctors pronouncing them dead and discover that they are out of their bodies. They notice that they are still in the same room and are observing the procedures of the medical team. The patients hear what is said, and they have difficulty believing that they are dead. They can see their lifeless bodies, but they feel fine. They notice "their bodies to be vacated as if it were a strange object" (Rawlings 1978, pp. 22,62).

Dr. Rawlings writes that people remember coming out of the body headfirst and floating over to the corner of the room or the ceiling, and they report looking down at their bodies. Clinically dead people try to inform their relatives that they are okay, but nobody can see them.

> The clinically dead person notices that he has a new body which is endowed with superior senses. He can go anywhere he wants and can read thoughts. He then moves through a tunnel. When he comes out of a tunnel he may see a beautiful environment. He meets and talks to friends and relatives who have previously died. He will see a being of light or a being of darkness. He may see a review of his life. He encounters some kind of a barrier and is turned back.

The soul goes to a good or bad place. The Greek philosopher Plato and also Socrates, the famous Athenian philosopher, taught the same phenomenon. I always had a feeling that we are dealing with two different entities, which are a soul and a spirit, in our lives.

I have been thinking about the distinction between the soul and the spirit for a long time because it is not explained well in literature. St. Thomas Aquinas said that the human soul is something incorporeal and subsistent, which means that it can survive. He also said that the soul can move.

Dr. Maurice Rawlings writes that all of his patients who reported a continuance from one life to another met their friends and relatives who have previously died in some kind of soothing place. They described being of light or being of darkness.

We believe only in what we can see, hear, feel, smell, and taste. Jesus knew that we are like this, and that is why he said that we do not see what we should see and do not hear what we should hear. The author also states that the Old Testament deals more with the resurrection, and the New Testament deals with everlasting life. Jesus told the repentant thief on the cross that he would be with him in paradise *today*. Dr. Rawlings further writes that for Christians, it is important to know that Christ said that because he lives; we shall live also (John 14:19).

Dr. Rawlings reports that patients confirmed both negative and positive experiences in equal numbers. People that had bad experiences during their clinical death described their experiences to Dr. Rawlings after they came back to life like this:

> Instead of emerging into bright surroundings they enter a dark, dim environment where they encounter grotesque people who may be lurking in the shadows or along a burning lake of fire. The horrors defy description and are difficult to recall. Compared to pleasant experiences, exact details are difficult to obtain. It is important to interview people who have died immediately upon resuscitation, while they are still in trouble and calling for help and before the experience can be forgotten or concealed. (Rawlings 1978, 63–64)

Dr. Rawlings noticed that bad experiences were very painful to the patient and therefore were removed from their conscious recall. Dr. Moody and Dr. Kübler-Ross, as well as other psychiatrists, interviewed patients several days or weeks after the date of their clinical death. In that time, the bad experiences were already forgotten (Rawlings 1978, 65–66).

Dr. Rawlings writes in his book a detailed report of a physician who, in 1889, was in a coma during a typhoid fever. He had died, and he watched the interesting process of separating soul and body. He recollected distinctly how he appeared to himself something like a jellyfish with regard to colour and form. His spirit then emerged, and he floated up and down until he at last broke loose from the body.

Then he slowly rose and extended to the full stature of a man. This was recorded in the November 1889 issue of the *St. Louis Medical and Surgical Journal* concerning Dr. Wiltse of Skiddy, Kansas, who was treated by a Dr. S.H. Raynes (Rawlings 1978, 68).

I wanted to write about the most interesting part of the story only, but the story is so persuading that I decided to write about the whole story. Recalling his own death, Dr. Wiltse reported that he seemed to be translucent of a bluish case, and as he turned to leave the room, his elbow came in contact with the arm of a gentleman who was standing in the door. To his surprise, his arm passed through Dr. Wiltse's without apparent resistance.

Dr. Rawlings writes that Dr. Wiltse described himself as being lifted and gently propelled through the air by someone's hands and placed on some road in the sky. He was aware of a presence that he could not see but which he knew was in the clouds. And as the cloud rested lightly upon either side of his head, the thoughts that entered his brain were not his thoughts. He was addressed kindly in his mother tongue so that he could understand, "All is well." He was also told that the road he was on was to the eternal world and that the rocks that he saw were the boundary between the two worlds and the two lives. He was told that if his work was complete on earth, he may pass beyond the rocks; but if it is not done, he could return to his body. He was tempted to cross the boundary line and stay. As he advanced, he was stopped, and he felt the power to move or to think was leaving him. The clouds touched his face, and he knew no more.

This is a historical example of life after death. The same report of Dr. Wiltse from the November 1889 issue of *The St. Louis Medical and Surgical Journal* was also reported in Dr. F.W.H. Myers book *Human Personality and Its Survival of Bodily Death*.

Another historical example of life after death that Dr. Rawlings wrote about involved a pioneer in psychoanalysis, Dr. Carl Gustav Jung. Jung describes what happened to him after a heart attack. He writes that after exiting his body, he found himself floating away from earth in a blue light, and he stood before a temple which had a door surrounded by a wreath of flames. He wrote that it is impossible to convey the beauty and intensity of emotions during his visions. He said that his experience was the most tremendous thing that had ever happened to him.

There is more written about Carl Jung's experiences in my notes from *Jung on Death and Immortality* written by Jenny Yates.

Dr. Rawlings describes variable experiences of his patients that died a clinical death in which the sequence of events is about the same, but some details of their experiences may be altered. It is difficult for a lot of patients to express what they saw. Many people encountered a barrier over which they could not pass and told us about it when they came back. Some people think that the place where they came may represent merely a sorting ground. Since people report good and bad experiences when they come back from a clinical death, we have to be careful while we are alive what kind of life we are living.

As mentioned before, people report that death itself is like a simple faint, a missed heartbeat, like going to sleep. People that had pleasant experiences are not afraid to die again. Dr. Rawlings mentions that some people think that there is no hell because God loves everybody. We know that Satan does not want to be identified and that he wants people to think that he doesn't exist.

People who had life-after-death experiences know that social status and wealth are not the most important things in life. Only love you show people will be remembered. People that died and had good experience are not afraid to die again. They talk about those people that are afraid of dying that they must have a reason. Dr. Rawlings mentioned in his book that the apostle Paul said that our bodies will be different when we come back to life. Those bodies will never die. Our bodies will be full of strength in our next life.

Many doctors who treated patients who have had near-death experiences describe what the patients told them after they were resuscitated back to life. Most of these people came to a beautiful place, but Dr. Rawlings writes also about people that describe themselves as having been in hell. Dr. Rawlings writes about Thomas Welch and his experience, described in his book *Oregon's Amazing Miracle*. In 1976, this publication was used with the author's permission. Thomas Welch writes that he was alive in another world. He fell over the edge of a trestle. The locomotive engineer watched him go down into the water. The next thing he could remember was standing near a shoreline of a great ocean of fire. He writes that there was no way to escape. He saw another man in front of him. It was Jesus. He wished he would rescue him from that place. Jesus looked at him, and Thomas Welch entered his body.

Thomas Welch asked God what he wanted him to do in his life. It was communicated to him to tell the world what he saw and how he came back to life.

In his book, Dr. Rawlings describes other experiences of his patients that report a hellish place. He said that variations in the figure that takes them away or sends them back from the spirit world seems to vary considerably among the bad experiences; but in the good experiences, it seems to be similar (Rawlings 1978, 107).

Many times in my life, I could not understand how people go through this life so self-satisfied, as though they would not have to face bad consequences. They like to hurt people. In our present lives, there is not much talk about the devil and hell. People were more aware about it in the olden days. I remember going to church when I was a little girl with my parents. The priests warned people about hell in a loud voice. You don't hear about it anymore in church today.

The patients who told their experiences to the doctors were convinced that there is life after death, and they are willing to dedicate their lives telling others about it. Dr. Rawlings writes that if there is a continuation of the spirit outliving the body, then we are talking about immortality. Some Protestant faiths prefer to believe that the spirit dies at the same time as the body and that both will be revived on the final day of the world. Dr. Rawlings writes only about what patients told him. He finds no reason to not believe that life after death occurs immediately after the spirit separates from the body. He mentions that Jesus taught that conscious existence continues after death and that there is a "good place" and a "bad place" prior to the final judgment.

The author writes that people believe that the universe is the result of the "big bang," an explosion of an original large mass of matter that created many smaller stars. But how can we find out where this original mass of matter came from? The next question is if there is a Creator who created the universe and life. Should we believe that everything came into existence from nothing?

We know that universe has an order, that it continues to obey precise physical laws. God shows us his love, but we don't see it. God gave us free will, but we use it to disobey him. God revealed himself through the prophets in the Old Testament and through his Son in the New Testament. We can learn about God by observing what he has created. People have made great scientific accomplishments, but they still do not know who God is.

Dr. Rawlings reminds us about the latest scientific observation. He mentions that the black hole, which is discharging deadly x-rays and has a tremendous gravitational pull such that is sucks up other stars and is increasing in size and mass, will eventually explode according to the astrophysicists. This may sound unbelievable to us, but it could actually be the truth (Rawlings 1978, 144). The author is asking the question if this is more ridiculous than saying that everything came into existence by itself. If God created all these billions of stars and planets, why did he love the earth so much? Life still appears to be unique to our planet. Why would God give the earth oxygen, chlorophyll, and water for maintaining life if he would not want to keep us for eternity? It remains a mystery why there is life on earth. We should also remember that God is still busy in the universe creating new stars and removing old ones (Psalm 102:25–26 and Hebrews 1:10–12). This is not only in the Bible, but science also talks about it (Rawlings 1978, 145).

I saw a documentary about stars in the universe, and it was also mentioned there. We think that we can understand everything, but we can't. We think that the science can explain how everything works, but it can't. Just read what I have found. Scientists don't know how to synthesize chlorophyll.

> Chlorophyll makes our food substances. In the presence of sunlight, it converts water and the carbon dioxide we exhale into starches and sugars. This starch from chlorophyll contained in the greens of all foliage and most produce, is the food of both man and animal…Bible suggests that only God can make it. Man admits he does not know how to make it. (Rawlings 1978, 147)

In my search of having the signs and messages from my husband explained, I have learned about different church doctrines. I was shocked that ministers of some Protestant churches still believe that both the body and the spirit die and will both resurrect at the end of the world, and yet they claim that they believe in Jesus Christ, that they live according to the Bible and they believe everything that is in the Bible. Which Bible? All the Bibles that I know talk about how Jesus died, that he was buried and was raised to life on the third day. He told the thief who was crucified beside him that he would be in paradise with him that same day! After his resurrection, Jesus appeared to many people such as Cephas, then to the twelve, and finally to five hundred of "the brothers" at the same time (1 Corinthians 15:3–8).

Many ministers of mainline churches are deviating from biblical teaching. "Satan, the Great Deceiver, is appearing in many areas of life as a false beam of light or as a prophet as a new lifestyle, leading many astray" (Rawlings 1978, 156). Many people treat church like a social club. We should know that this is not enough. We should all try to acquire the knowledge about life after death. This will encourage us to live a life in such a way that we will be better people and won't be afraid to die. It is very disappointing to know that some ministers of some Christian denominations are leading their congregations astray by telling them that they are teaching them according to the Bible, and it is not true. Jesus died for us so that we could have an everlasting life that will begin right away when we die and not at the end of the world. He has demonstrated it himself by his resurrection and by appearing to so many people after his death. We can learn all about it from the Bible.

Life at Death: A Scientific Investigation of the Near-Death Experience

Dr. Kenneth Ring

After I read *Life at Death* by Kenneth Ring, the first scientific investigation of near-death experiences, I felt a huge relief. I felt confident that what I have experienced is worth telling to the public. From interviews with more than a hundred men and women who have experienced clinical death, Dr. Ring shows that certain elements are common. Dr. Ring calls the typical near-death experience the "core experience." Clinical death is a state in which vital signs such as heartbeats and respiration are entirely absent. Dr. Ring confirms the findings reported by Dr. Raymond Moody in his book *Life after Life*.

Dr. Ring questioned if science can explain by itself near-death experiences. According to him, near-death experiences may have a nonphysical quality.

Dr. Kenneth Ring interviewed 102 patients. Forty-nine had near-death experiences. He mentioned in his book *Life at Death* that he has studied near-death experiences only. The people that he interviewed were clinically dead but were resuscitated and came back to life. He was asked many times if he thinks that there is life after death. This is what he said:

> I do believe…that we continue to have a conscious existence after our physical death and that the core experience does represent its beginning, a glimpse of things to come. I am, in fact, convinced—both from my own personal experiences and from my studies as a psychologist—that it is possible to become conscious of "other realities" and that the coming close to death represents one avenue to a higher "frequency domain," or reality, which will be fully accessible to us following what we call death. (Ring 1980, 254–255)

Dr. Kenneth Ring regards near-death experiences as "teachings." These experiences, according to him, clearly imply that there is something more, something beyond the physical world of the senses that is a greater spectrum of reality. To the question why such experiences occur, Dr. Ring had a speculative answer:

> I have come to believe that the universe (if I may put it in this fashion) has many ways of "getting its message across." In a sense, it wants us to "wake up" to become aware of the cosmic dimensions of the drama of which we are all a part. Near-death experiences represent one of its devices for waking us up to this higher reality. The "message"—for the experiencing individuals at least—is usually so clear, potent, and undeniable that it is neither forgotten nor dismissed. Potentially, then those who have these experiences become "prophets" to the rest of us. (Ring 1980, 255)

Near-death experiences are nothing new. A talk about death is a "taboo," even if death is a part of our living on this earth. We have a promise to live forever. Why shouldn't we educate ourselves about it and get prepared? We work so hard to make our life here on earth better, even if it is just for a short time, but we don't think about eternity. People are scared to talk about death. We don't have to be scared to die. My husband died with great dignity. He never complained about his condition. When I started to talk about his problems, he told me to be positive. He told a patient, a priest, that he was going to die and that he was ready. He did not stay home to feel sorry for himself; he was working until the last day. Before we took him to the hospital, I could see that he didn't feel well, and I told him to stay home. He told me, "The patients need me."

Dr. Ring knows how concerned people are about the destiny of the human race on this planet. After Dr. Ring finished his research, he was happy in that respect that his findings corresponded with findings of other studies. He felt that more studies were necessary. In the conclusion of his book, he wrote:

> Too much of our data comes from ex post facto accounts and, correspondingly, not enough from on-the-scene witnesses. Such investigations are particularly crucial to assessing such notions as a Rawlings' repression hypothesis and the hypothesis that the double separates from the physical body at death. (Ring 1980, 259)

Dr. Ring had in mind the establishment of a facility where terminally ill individuals would live while being prepared to die with full awareness of the transcendent potentialities inherent in the process of dying. He writes that many researchers such as Moody, Kübler-Ross, Osis, and others have established a pattern showing that these experiences eliminate the fear of death from the patients. They also agree on the pattern that these patients experience a "profoundly beautiful transformation in consciousness." These people are "prepared to face death fearlessly and joyously" (Ring 1980, 280).

Dr. Ring believes survivors of near-death experiences can teach us all how to live. Dr. Ring believed that his investigation represents the most systematic and exhaustive scientific study of near-death experiences thus far reported. People that had the core experience usually keep their experience for themselves because they are afraid that people will not understand. They fear that they will be disbelieved or ridiculed. I can compare this to my experience with the signs and messages from my husband. By talking to about 250 people about it, I have found out that people have had similar experiences themselves or knew about someone who received them. Also, they told me about it only in exchange for my information. This area of knowledge is still very much taboo. I know that I can anticipate little support from the sceptical world in which we are living, but I know that the people that told me about their experiences with this phenomenon—and that was almost all the people I talked to about it—will believe me. I took the phone numbers of those people, and I will try to phone them after my book will be published. Most of them were my husband's patients. These people were very supportive of my idea to do some research and write a book about it, including my own experiences. My husband's patients want to know what their doctor's message is, and they are among those people to whom I dedicate my book. They know me and trust me.

In his investigation into the near-death experiences, Dr. Ring reports very similar findings as those of other studies undertaken by other doctors. At the out-of-body stage, the respondents tended to claim that their thinking processes were clear and sharp, logical, and were governed by rational rather than emotional considerations. They felt no anxiety, were relaxed, completely calm. They could see and hear at first, but later on they existed as "mind only." Patients first experience peace and well-being, which soon turns into joy and happiness. The individual may experience buzzing or a wind-like sound, and he finds himself looking down on his physical body. His vision and hearing tends to be more acute than usual. He is aware of the actions and conversations taking place in the physical environment. He feels being drawn into another reality. Dr. Ring writes that the patients experienced many of the same things that previous studies had found: a presence, floating through a tunnel, a review of the person's life, reuniting with one's deceased loved ones, and a decision must be made to live or die (Ring 1980, 102–103).

The Cell's Design: How Chemistry Reveals the Creator's Artistry

Fazale Rana, PhD

It was very difficult for me to read and to write about Dr. Rana's *The Cell's Design*. I wanted to reveal God to people who will read my book because I know that they should first believe in God if they should believe in the afterlife. In his book, Dr. Rana reveals God; and therefore, I had to include his book in my research. Dr. Rana writes about what contemporary science had learned about the cell's design, and he shows that it is the work of an intelligent Designer, the God of the Scriptures. He is letting us know how the cell was designed and that there is evidence of a Designer.

Dr. Rana stated that 150 years ago, after Darwin's publication of *On the Origin of Species*, the living cell was thought to be something that has evolved: a microscopic blob of gelatine. New discoveries in science now show how complicated the cell is. We know now that the cell is too complex and could not have just happened. The complexity of cell design is something that naturalism cannot explain. There is a universal recognition that biochemical systems appear to be designed. Dr. Rana confesses that

> this elegance, evident in virtually all aspects of the cell's chemistry, carries a profound philosophical and theological

significance that prompts questions about the origin, purpose, and meaning of life. Though I once embraced the evolutionary paradigm, its inadequate explanations for the origin of life, coupled with the sophistication and complexity of the cell's chemical systems convinced me as a biochemistry graduate student that a Creator must exist. (Rana 2008, 17)

Recent advances in biochemistry reveal biochemical systems that seem far more purposeful, intricate, and sophisticated than ever imagined, writes Dr. Rana. Dr. Rana mentions that in his book *Darwin's Black Box*, Michael Behe argues that biochemical systems, by their very nature, are irreducibly complex. Dr. Rana mentions that, according to Behe, irreducible complexity is described as "a single system composed of several well-matched, interacting parts that contribute to the basic function, wherein the removal of any one of the parts causes the system to effectively cease functioning" (Rana 2008, 18). Dr. Rana writes that *Darwin's Black Box* emphasizes the inability of natural selection to generate irreducibly complex systems in a gradual stepwise evolutionary process. He mentions that irreducible complexity is but one of the biochemical features that point to intelligent design. Dr. Rana can see in the cell a supernatural basis for life. He mentions that if we are to believe that evolutionary biologists are telling us the truth, they have to explain in detail how biochemical systems originated all on their own. They have to consider that astronomers tell us that there is not enough time or resources throughout the universe's history to generate life in its simplest form. According to Dr. Rana,

> various lines of evidence can also make a powerful case that life's molecular artistry stems from the Creator described in the Bible. To be convincing, this position must be built upon a weight of evidence. For an idea to gain credibility in the scientific arena, it must find support from a

collective body of data that works in concert to support one conclusion. (Rana 2008, 32)

Dr. Rana can see in the biochemical systems specified complexity that results from forethought and planning. He reminds us that we can know about God from what he has done. Dr. Rana mentions that if life has a supernatural origin, then the cells are the work of a Creator. The cells are very complex. By reducing the complexity of the cell, the cell would stop functioning. The cell can work only by the way it was designed. Dr. Rana writes about the theory that states that cells are the fundamental units of life and the smallest entities that can be considered "life" (Rana 2008, 36).

In his book, Dr. Rana provides a description of the cell and its molecular constituents. Dr. Rana mentions that biochemist Michael Behe argues that individual biochemical systems are irreducibly complex, and so is life itself. Behe makes the powerful case that irreducibly complex systems cannot emerge through an undirected stepwise process. Behe argues how the incredibly complex nature of minimal life makes it difficult to envision how natural evolutionary processes could have produced even the simplest life-form. Dr. Rana and astronomer Hugh Ross, the author of *Origins of Life*, reached the identical conclusion that if left up to an evolutionary process, not enough resources or time exists throughout the universe's history to generate life in its simplest form. In his book, Dr. Rana shows that there are little motors visible in the cells that resemble those designed by humans. It illustrates that God designed these motors first during his creation and that the cell's machinery indicates that life's chemistry stems from an intelligent agency. "The molecular motors are irreducibly complex, an independent indicator of intelligent design" (Rana 2008, 96). Dr. Rana also writes,

> The cell's machinery is vastly superior to anything that the best human designers can conceive or accomplish…The

superiority of the cell's molecular machines is consistent with the notion that an intelligent designer is the Creator described in the Bible. (Rana 2008, 87)

Evolutionary biologists have to prove that this irreducibly complex system has an evolutionary origin by providing a detailed description of the evolutionary process. They also have to demonstrate that this process could have happened in the available time and available resources during the evolution. (Rana, 2008, p. 272)

Dr. Rana not only shows us pictures of molecular motors but also other molecular structures in the cell in his book *The Cell's Design*. His book shows the scientific and theological importance of what was discovered. He is pointing at biochemical features that can help us believe in the Creator.

The Spiritual Doorway in the Brain: A Neurologist's Search for the God Experience

KEVIN NELSON, MD

This book is different in the respect that it is trying to explain near-death experiences from the point of a living brain, which is a completely different approach from the other scientific investigations of doctors that I have researched before, including Dr. Wilder Penfield, who had also studied a living human brain together with the brains of clinically dead people. Dr. Kevin Nelson is talking about the mind as being something of a brain mechanism (Nelson 2011, 50). Dr. Wilder Penfield operated on many brains, and he could see that the brain is not capable of the usual functions during clinical deaths. Dr. Penfield also helped us solve the puzzle of how people can see during clinical deaths. He talked to people who had died and came back. He found that we have the soul and the mind and that the mind has energy (Penfield 1975, *The Mystery of the Mind*, p. 48). The comparison of the research of Dr. Kevin Nelson and Dr. Wilder Penfield is very important. Dr. Kevin Nelson believes that it is through the brain that people see during their clinical death in comparison to Dr. Wilder Penfield, who proved in his research that it is impossible to see what people see during their clinical death with their brain (Penfield 1975, 85–90).

The experiences of people that described what they saw were based on clinical death, where their brains did not function. The brain could resume its function only with the help of the lungs and the heart after the resuscitation process. Dr. Kevin Nelson's observations are based on the study of a functional and live brain. A healthy brain can't be compared to a brain that is not functional.

Research of near-death experiences are done all over the world. These researchers reported many common features. Dr. Kevin Nelson tried to explain near-death experiences in terms of a REM sleep, even if other scientists had shown that the brain does not dream during clinical deaths. What people saw during their clinical deaths was clear, not distorted like in dreams. If people couldn't remember dreams while they were healthy, how could they remember so clearly when they were clinically dead? Even if Dr. Kevin Nelson believed that there might be a spiritual doorway in the brain, the fact is that the brain had been dead for a few minutes and didn't function until the resuscitation process revived it. And without the function of the heart and the lungs, the brain would not be able to resume this function.

In my research, I was also trying to understand theology to see how God fits into this life-after-death phenomenon. Because scientists in general are atheists, it is very difficult for them to understand and to explain what is going on during near-death experiences. Only with the help of theology can they see that they can't explain scientifically what is going on. Many scientists started to believe in God after they saw that the scientific explanations are failing. Dr. Kevin Nelson also writes in his book, "To me faith and science are not as different as some people have made them" (Nelson 2011, 259). Since the scientists can't find the nature of near-death experiences, researchers agree that the mind exists separate from the physical brain. For Dr. Kevin Nelson, such a claim is the most extraordinary in all of science. How much more can science do to explain these experiences? It looks like science can't explain the unexplainable in the terms of science, but theology can explain it in terms of theology.

The Language of God: A Scientist Presents Evidence for Belief

Dr. Francis S. Collins

I have chosen Dr. Francis S. Collins's book *The Language of God* for my research even if it does not have anything to do with life after death because I know that to believe in the afterlife means to believe in God. Dr. Collins's belief in a Designer, God, that made earth and all the living things on it is empowering. His conversion from being an atheist to a believer in God is described so well in his book *The Language of God* that I am wondering how an atheist could resist Dr. Collins's enthusiasm for God and his work. His explanation of evolution is the best I have ever heard of. He explains the misunderstanding of evolution portrayed to us by Darwin in a way that is logical and easy to understand. As a girl of about twelve or thirteen years old, I was taught at school in communist Czechoslovakia that evolution happens only within the species and that one species never evolves into another species. I never forgot about that. I never thought about it until I went to Canada and heard from my children how evolution is taught in schools here. It was upsetting to me, but I could not change my children's education. Because I was put into the position of the author of a book that I truly care for, I had to establish my ground. I had to do it for everybody who will read my book.

Dr. Collins's book made a tremendous impression on me. I wish that everybody would read his book. In it, Dr. Collins talks about his wonder when he found out how a man was made and about his belief that man had to be designed. The fact is that for a man to be designed, there was a need of a designer. Dr. Collins writes, "Life appears designed so there must be a designer" (Collins 2006, 148). There is no need for a designer in a theory of evolution. I am surprised how many people today still believe all that the theory of evolution claims. Some of the authors of the books that I have read for my research agree that there is a unity of knowledge between faith and science. Science teaches us to understand the natural world and material existence, but not the spiritual world.

According to Dr. Collins, there is no conflict in being a scientist and a person who believes in God. In Dr. Collins's words, "Science's domain is to explain nature. God's domain is in the spiritual world, a realm not possible to explore with the tools and the language of science. It must be explained with the heart, the mind and the soul and the mind must find a way to embrace both realms" (Collins 2006, 6). Dr. Collins, the director of the Human Genome Project, contributed a great deal to our understanding of the human genome. He explains DNA as God's instruction book of science and the work of a Designer. Dr. Collins is a man of faith, and he sees God as a Creator while reflecting on the relationship between faith and science. In his book *The Language of God*, he writes how complex the information within each cell of the human body is. He believes that science is the only reliable way to understand the natural world, but it can't answer the spiritual questions. We all want to know if there is life after death. Science can't find out.

Dr. Collins writes that we blame God for our suffering, but it was humans who invented instruments like arrows, knives, guns, and bombs that torture us. He mentions that the tragedies caused by the use of their instruments can't be blamed upon God as God gave us free will. People use free will to disobey the moral law instilled in us by God, argues Dr. Collins. He states that we should not blame natural disasters on God and explain it with the words of the Anglican priest and distinguished physicist John Polkinghorn, who referred to these categories of events as "physical evil," as opposed to the moral evil committed by humankind (Collins 2006, 43–45).

Dr. Collins writes that science reveals the evolutionary process of the universe, our own planet, and the life on it. This process can include changes in the weather, the slippage of a tectonic plate, or the misspelling of a cancer gene in the process of cell division, showing that God's plans may not be the same as our plans. Dr. Collins realizes that people are growing and learning through suffering and that this knowledge is universal in the world's great faiths. According to Buddha, "Life is suffering." Dr. Collins thinks that for the believer, this realization can be a source of great comfort (Collins 2006, 47). Dr. Collins was one of the scientists working on decoding DNA, which he calls "the language of God." When Dr. Collins started to study DNA, he was astounded. He felt a desire to contribute something to humanity, so he applied for admission to medical school and was overwhelmed by the amazing complexity of the human body. He saw that it was not just the cell that provides a source of wonder but the entire organism. He was astounded by the elegance of the human DNA code and the multiple consequences and the rare careless moments of its copying mechanism causing disorders, some from merely a single letter gone awry (Collins 2006, 18).

Dr. Collins participated in the Human Genome Project, one of the most historic undertakings of humankind. Six months into the new millennium, humankind crossed a bridge into the momentous new era when the first draft of the human genome, our own instruction book, had been assembled (Collins 2006, 1). The Human Genome Project is one of the major achievements of humankind. There were more than two thousand scientists who accomplished the project.

Dr. Collins was the project manager. Dr. Collins further writes that the human genome consists of all the DNA of our species, the hereditary code of life (Collins 2006, 17). This script contains all the instructions for building a human being that was previously known only to God. To understand the questions that most of us have about the universe, human existence, and the afterlife, we have to look for answers in science and in religion. The meaning of human existence, the existence of God, and the possibility of an afterlife that I am trying to understand through my research lie outside the scientific method. Human beings have questions, and they want to find the answers to what is seen as well as what is unseen. Dr. Collins is giving us an opportunity to look for answers. He mentions that God is not threatened by science because he made science possible. With the help of the teachings of C.S. Lewis, the legendary Oxford scholar who used to be an atheist, Dr. Collins learned about the "moral law." Dr. Collins mentions that human beings are breaking the moral law all the time and seem unable to live up to it. Dr. Collins knows that the search for God is universal. He thinks that the search is the human longing, which he hopes has a chance for fulfillment. Because of this longing, he thinks that people should know that they were made for another world.

We can't find out how our world and everything else on it was created. Dr. Collins writes, "I cannot see how nature could have created itself. Only a supernatural force that is outside of space and time could have done it" (Collins 2006, 67). Dr. Collins mentions that the opening words of Genesis state that in the beginning, God created the heavens and the earth, which is compatible with the big bang. The big bang theory is what science tells us (Collins 2006, 150). All of this means that God existed before he created the heavens and the earth and that the big bang theory points to the Creator (Collins 2006, 77).

Humans have a particular interest in the fossil records of our species, but their puzzles are yet to be solved. I will talk a little about the fossil records of humans only because it is connected with what I want people to know—that to believe in life after death, they first should believe in God and that he is our Creator. Dr. Collins writes that a dozen different hominid species have been discovered in Africa, which shows a steadily increasing cranial capacity. "The specimen we recognize as modern homo sapiens date from about 195000 years ago" (Collins 2006, 96).

In order to be able to write about what I think people should know, I have to write about Charles Darwin. Charles Darwin believed in his theory of evolution, which claims that one species can evolve into another species, but there are only changes within species visible. Darwin claims that we have evolved from a small set of ancestors, perhaps just one. Darwin talks about it in his book *The Descent of Man*. According to the theory of evolution, our closest living relatives are the *chimpanzees*. Humans and chimps are 96 percent identical at the DNA level. A further examination of human and chimpanzee chromosomes showed the difference between humans and chimpanzees. "The human has twenty-three pairs of chromosomes, but the chimpanzee has twenty-four" (Collins 2006, 137). There is a proposition that "evolution is fundamentally flawed, since it cannot account for the intricate complexity of nature" (Collins 2006, 184).

Dr. Collins writes that the study of genomes shows that humans share a common ancestor with other living things, but it does not prove a common ancestor. Dr. Collins thinks that this evidence could demonstrate that God used successful design principles over and over again. Comparing human and mouse genes, for example, shows the same order, but the spacing in between the genes is different (Collins 2006, 134). At the DNA level, we humans are all 99.9 percent identical. "By DNA analysis, we humans are truly part of one family." This applies to all individuals from around the world. Population geneticists conclude that we humans have descended from a common set of fenders (Collins 2006, 125–126). Some critics of Darwinism argue that there is no evidence of major changes in species in the fossil record, only change within species. They have not seen new species arise (Collins 2006, 131–132). One hundred and fifty years after Darwin's publication of *On the Origin of Species*, the public controversy about evolution has not been resolved yet (Collins 2006, 158).

As a geneticist, biologist, and a believer in God, Dr. Collins is amazed by the molecular machines that reside in the inner working of the cell. In his book *The Language of God*, Dr. Collins cites a biochemist and a professor of biology, Michael Behe, who in his book *Darwin's Black Box* argues that "machines of this sort could never have arisen on the basis of natural selection." Behe mentions that the whole arrangement in the cell is an engineering marvel (Collins 2006, 185). Dr. Collins was converted from being an atheist to a believer in God, whom he saw as the Designer of all the complexity of life.

Many people wonder about the timing of the creation of the earth and the life on it. Some people insist upon a completely literal interpretation of Genesis, including twenty-four-hour days. St. Augustine questions the duration of the seven days of biblical creation. He writes, "What kind of days these were it is extremely difficult or perhaps impossible for us to conceive" (Collins 2006, 152). St. Augustine mentions in his work that God is outside of time and not bounded by it. He also mentioned that in the Bible, Peter states, "With the Lord a day is like a thousand years, and a thousand years are like a day" (2 Peter 3:8). These questions were debated by different people for centuries (Collins 2006, 151).

Dr. Collins searched to confirm the authenticity of Jesus Christ, who claimed that he is the Son of God. He found that all that is written in the New Testament about Jesus Christ is true. Dr. Collins was surprised at the historical evidence of the existence of Jesus Christ according to the historical books that he examined. The Gospels of Matthew, Mark, Luke, and John were written just a few decades after Christ's death, and their style and content suggests they are the record of eyewitnesses (Collins 2006, 223). Dr. Collins first thought that there could be errors made by successive copying or bad translation, but early manuscripts showed the evidence of authenticity of the four Gospels. Dr. Collins has once again stressed that science is the only way to investigate the natural world and natural events, but science can't explain human existence, God, and the possibility of an afterlife, which people want so desperately to know. The cooperation of science and religion is needed to make new discoveries.

He mentions that even Albert Einstein saw the importance of science and religion when he wrote, "Science without religion is lame, religion without science is blind" (Collins 2006, 228).

It looks like God wants us to know about him, and therefore, he lets our departed loved ones to let us know that they are not really dead, only transformed into a different kind of being. Why else would they let us know that they exist? I know that the signs our departed loved ones are showing we are difficult to understand. It is also difficult for me, and that is why I did the research. I talked to a monk about what happened to me and my family, and he told me that deceased people are allowed by God to do it. All this shows us that God wants us to know that he exists and that there is an afterlife. He knows that it is hard for us to understand it, but we have more knowledge about him and his creation now than before, and we should try to learn about him. The knowledge of people like Dr. Collins about God's work is very valuable to us. I hope that in the future there will be even more knowledge about God and his work available to us.

Quantum Physics and Theology: An Unexpected Kinship

John Polkinghorne

John Polkinghorne spent a long time working as a theoretical physicist, and later on he studied theology and was ordained to the Anglican priesthood. In science and in theology, he was searching for the truth. In his book *Quantum Physics and Theology: An Unexpected Kinship*, John Polkinghorne makes comparisons between modern quantum physics and understanding of God. He is interested in both science and theology because they are both concerned with the search for truth. According to him, science and theology complement each other rather than contrast each other. He writes, "Of course, the two disciplines focus on different dimensions of truth, but they share a common conviction that there is truth to be sought" (Polkinghorne 2007, 1). John Polkinghorne not only solved my problem with understanding why these two words got into my thoughts or mind—namely, the words *quantum mechanics*—but he also strengthened my belief that Jesus Christ is the Son of God.

In his book, he writes about the differences between theology and science. John Polkinghorne writes that the same as there is quantum faith, there is a Christian faith. Certain phenomena are impossible to explain with science, and certain phenomena are impossible to explain in theology. Richard Feynman wrote about quantum mechanics this way:

> Because atomic behavior is so unlike ordinary experience, it is very difficult to get used to, and it appears peculiar and mysterious to everyone…We shall tackle immediately the basic element of the mysterious behavior in its most strange form. We choose to examine a phenomenon which is impossible, absolutely impossible, to explain in any classical way and which has in it the heart of quantum mechanics. (Polkinghorne 2007, 18–19)

In quantum science, there are still matters that scientists don't understand, and they can't explain what they need to explain. The same as scientists have problems explaining the physical world, the writers of the New Testament had a problem with both human and divine qualities of Jesus Christ. John Polkinghorne writes:

> If Jesus was just an unusually inspired man, the use of the divine language of lordship about Him would seem to have been an unfortunate error, quite inappropriate for someone who was simply a human being, however remarkable. The first Christians testified to the experience of a new power at work in their lives. Something must have happened to continue the story of Jesus. Whatever it was must have been of a magnitude adequate to explain the transformation that came on His followers, changing that bunch of frightened deserters who ran away when he was arrested; into those who would face the authorities in Jerusalem…what had happened was the resurrection of Jesus from the dead on the third day after his execution. (Polkinghorne 2007, 32–39)

The Bible speaks about appearances occurring over a forty-day period. John Polkinghorne believes that the appearance stories demand to be taken very seriously as well as the finding of the empty tomb. Both are the evidence of the truth of the resurrection of Jesus.

There is no suggestion anywhere of Jesus being buried a second time. The author states that, according to Jewish custom, after a corpse had been in the tomb for about a year, been reduced to a skeleton, the bones are usually taken away and placed in an ossuary for interment elsewhere. Nothing like this happened to Jesus. John Polkinghorne believes that was because there were no bones to be dealt with (Polkinghorne 2007, 46).

John Polkinghorne writes that using Aramaic *Cephas* for Peter and the reference to the apostles as "the twelve" shows the integrity of the writings in the four Gospels. There was good evidence that Jesus was raised from the dead. According to John Polkinghorne, there are two reasons to consider. The first reason is the Christian establishment of Sunday as the Lord's Day in place of the Jewish Sabbath, which was established to commemorate his day of rising. The second reason is that Jesus is always mentioned as the living Lord in the present, not in the past.

John Polkinghorne sees a perfect union of God and man in the incarnation on which the whole Christian life depends. According to Polkinghorne, God has purpose for people on earth. God had installed a moral law into humans, which human beings seem to be incapable to keep.

This book was very important for me to read. It explained to me why the two words *quantum mechanics* were put into my mind. It showed me that if quantum mechanics cannot be totally explained, the soul and near-death experiences couldn't be totally explained. Science, the same as theology, has many unexplainable areas that neither scientists nor theologians can explain and probably will never be able to explain. John Polkinghorn's book taught me that I can't explain unexplainable; I can only try to understand it. According to Polkinghorne, there is a relationship between faith and science. Science and theology have to cooperate so that new scientific discoveries can be made.

John Polkinghorne is still trying to find the truth in both science and theology.

People depend on science to explain everything that they want to be explained but often can't find the explanation. Even with Darwin's help, science can't explain the origin of life on Earth. Darwin's theory of natural selection can never explain the complexity of life on earth. The Bible doesn't deny the big bang and teaches us in Genesis that God created the world. The New Testament is credible because people who knew Jesus and witnessed what he did wrote it. There is wisdom in all God's laws. God gave us a free will, but we have to obey His laws. We are responsible for our own actions. We have to stop trying to change the nature, change the crops, and polluting the earth; all that is against God's laws. God wants us to love one another. We have to try to stop the wars.

The Philosophical Writings of Descartes, Volume I and II

TRANSLATED BY JOHN COTTINGHAM, ROBERT STOOTHOFF, AND DUGALD MURDOCH

*D*escartes was born on March 31, 1596. In his early writings, Descartes describes God as pure intelligence. He said, "The Lord has made three marvels: something out of nothing; free will; and God in man" (Cottingham, Dugald, and Stoothoff 1985, 5). In his "Rules for the Direction of the Mind: Rule One" in his *The Philosophical Writings of Descartes*, Descartes mentions that people think that each science should be studied separately without regard to any of the others, but he does not think so. He thinks that all the sciences are closely interconnected and interdependent. By reading Descartes's work, I was surprised at how knowledgeable he was about different sciences and disciplines. It was always his most earnest desire to learn to distinguish truth from falsehood.

Descartes was fascinated with the human body, the machine made by the hands of God from the earth by which he meant the "elements" and which exhibits more artistry than anybody can possibly ascribe to it. He noticed that because the person can notice that he exists, the person is thinking. Descartes noticed that this "I" is the soul by which I am what I am and that this soul is entirely distinct from the body and is easier to know than the body. Descartes recognized that the intellectual part of a person is distinct from the corporal. He writes, "Our soul is of a nature entirely independent of the body, and consequently that it is not bound to die with it. And since we cannot see any other causes which destroy the soul, we are naturally led to conclude that it is immortal" (Cottingham, Dugald, and Stoothoff 1985, 141).

Descartes believed that the soul can exist independently of the body, which supports the scientific findings of Dr. Parnia and Dr. Sabom. If the soul can exist independently and if the mind has a nonphysical energy, then my husband's soul can travel and be with me any time he wants. This explains to me the signs he gave me and my children. The scientific experiments of Dr. Parnia and Dr. Sabom have proven that what people see when they are clinically dead has nothing to do with their brain because the brain is not functioning. It must, therefore, be the soul that gets out of the body at the time of death.

In his writings about God, Descartes tells us to remember that God is infinite, and we are finite. Descartes wants us to bear in mind that God is the Creator of all things. God, being infinite, means that he has no limits. He is great in excellence and is boundless and perfect—the infinite being. He is the Almighty in comparison to us, who, being finite, are subject to limitations or conditions. We are subject to the laws of nature, time, and circumstances; we are limited. It always amazes me how few people really know that God is almighty and how we, in comparison to him, are limited and therefore should be humble. If people would realize this limitation, then it would be easier for them to believe that God gave us a soul that is immortal. In order to be immortal, the soul can't die. If the soul can't die, there must be an afterlife. If the soul doesn't die and exists, God could allow the soul to let the soul's loved ones to know that it exists. If people accept that God is almighty, it would help them understand what God reveals to us. Descartes writes:

> Hence, if God happens to reveal to us something about Him or others which is beyond the natural reach of our mind—such as the mystery of the incarnation or of the trinity—we will not refuse to believe it, despite the fact that we do not clearly understand it. And we will not be at all surprised that there is much, both in the immeasurable nature of God and in the things created by Him, which is beyond our mental capacity. (Cottingham, Dugald, and Stoothoff 1985, 201)

The brains of our human bodies are limited. They don't work with full capacity, and God did not reveal to us the whole truth about himself. Many people think that what we know about God is all that there is. I am sure that God has plans for the world, and therefore, we should not be so arrogant to try to share in God's plans. But I am afraid that we are doing it. Descartes was one of the world's greatest philosophers. He was also a scientist. He believed in God, and he believed that we have a soul that is immortal. "Since the mind is by nature different from the body and from the disposition of the body, and cannot arise from this disposition, it is incorruptible" (Cottingham, Dugald, and Stoothoff 1985, 295). Descartes also writes about the mind and soul this way: "The mind has two different sorts of thought: intellect and volition" (Cottingham, Dugald, and Stoothoff 1985, 296).

> But when we try to get to know our nature more distinctly we can see that our soul, in so far as it is a substance which is distinct from the body, is known to us merely through the fact that it thinks, that is to say, understands, wills, imagines, remembers and has sensory perceptions; for all these functions are kinds of thought. (Cottingham, Dugald, and Stoothoff 1985, 314)

Thus, Descartes writes, are the actions that depend on the soul. Descartes believed that the soul could exist without the body. "And accordingly, it is certain that I (that is, my soul, by which I am what I am), am really distinct from my body, and can exist without it" (Cottingham, Dugald, and Stoothoff 1985, 54).

Republic

PLATO

Plato was born in Athens in 427 BC and died in 347 BC. He was born into a wealthy and prominent family. He was deeply affected by the condemnation and execution of his master Socrates (469–399 BC) on charges of irreligion and corrupting the young. When he was about forty years old, Plato founded the academy. The most celebrated member was young Aristotle (384–322 BC), who studied there for the last twenty years of Plato's life. Their works mark the highest peak of philosophical achievement in antiquity, and both continue to rank among the greatest philosophers of all time. Plato is the earliest Western philosopher from whose complete works have been preserved (from *Oxford World's Classics*). Plato joined the circle of followers of Socrates, and Socrates became the philosophical influence on Plato's life and thinking. Socrates was a great individualist and was killed for promoting individualism and therefore subverting the traditional state-centered values, and it is clear that Plato inherited this tendency from his master (from *Republic*, "*Introduction*"). He was a proponent of morality, and he was trying to show that the major cause of happiness is morality. He was trying to prove that anyone who is moral is better off than anyone who is not. The author also talks at the end of the book that morality is assimilation to God. Plato wanted his readers to change their lives to the image of God.

RESEARCH INTO THE AFTERLIFE

I have chosen to read Plato's *Republic* mainly because I was surprised to find that someone who was living from 427–347 BC was describing God in our modern terms despite of the fact that, in his time, Greeks had all kinds of Gods. I also knew that he wrote in his *Republic* about the soldier by the name of Er and described what Er saw when he had his near-death experience. In short, Plato's vision is of a rationally ordered universe, where everything has its place and its purpose. This vision of the order is shown in the myth of Er with which the book concludes. The point is that according to Plato, the universe is good because it is rationally ordered. Plato seems to suggest "as above, so below." Plato stresses the importance of goodness. According to Plato, goodness is related to morality.

In his book *Republic*, Plato is also talking about the mind. He thinks that its association with the body and with other evils can deform the mind. Plato is trying to see what the mind is like when the mind is untainted. He states that the mind is attracted toward wisdom and that we should consider that it is of the same order as the divine, immortal, and eternal realm. In Plato's time, the problem in Greek popular ethics was that it was known that immoral people's external affairs often appeared to prosper while those of moral people suffer. Plato's response to this is that a moral person has God's favor and will eventually prosper while an immoral person will sooner or later suffer catastrophe (Waterfield 2008, 368). Finally, according to Plato, morality also brings rewards after death. In his book *Republic*, Plato depicts the horrors of the punishments that await an immoral person in Hades. The myth about Er emphasizes order in one's mind, which is morality. There is a belief that Plato used this literary form because he believed in all the ingredients of the myth. Plato tells the story of the brave Er in his book *Republic* this way:

> Once upon a time, he was killed in battle, and by the time the corpses were collected, ten days later, they had all putrefied except his, which was still in good shape. He was taken home

and twelve days after his death, just as his funeral was about to start and he was lying on the pyre, he came back to life. Then he told people what he'd seen in the other world. He said that his soul left his body and went on a journey, with lots of other souls as his companions. They came to an awesome place, where they found two openings next to each other in the earth and two others directly opposite them up in the sky. There were judges sitting between the openings who made their assessment and then told the moral ones to take the right-hand route which went up and through the sky... but told the immoral ones to take the left-hand downward route....When Er approached, however, the judges said that he had to report back to mankind about what goes on there, and they told him to listen and observe everything that happened in the place. (Waterfield 2008, 371–372)

It is interesting to note that Plato believed in the afterlife and in Er's description of the penalties and punishments and the equivalent rewards. Plato believed in heaven and hell similarly as most people believe today. Plato finishes his book *Republic* with these words:

Anyway, my recommendation would be for us to regard the soul as immortal and as capable of surviving a great deal of suffering, just as it survives all the good times. We should always keep to the upward path, and we should use every means at our disposal to act morally and with intelligence, so that we may gain our own and the god's approval, not only during our stay here on earth. (Waterfield 2008, 379)

By reading about Plato, I learned that he also believed in separation of the soul, which is in the physical body only until the death of the body. At death, the soul separates from the body and continues to live in eternity.

Life after Death: The Burden of Proof

Dr. Deepak Chopra

*E*verybody agrees that life is a mystery, and eternal life is yet another mystery. Scientists are trying hard to explain how life originated, and theologians, along with scientists, are trying hard to find out about eternal life. Quantum theory fails to explain the origin of life and eternal life. Will the in-development new theory be more helpful to explain any of the two mysteries? I doubt it. I was never interested in any of the two mysteries; I just took them for granted until my husband died. He was a very clever man dedicated to his family and his patients, and I know that he was trying very hard to let me know that we don't really die, that we just cross over. Dr. Chopra is trying to explain an eternal mystery his own way. What I have found out from the books that I have researched is that life on earth begins with birth and ends with death while life in eternity begins with the change of the life-form. The soul lives another life that is not known to us. We learn about the life in eternity through the help of people that died a clinical death and came back to life and through the help of the departed souls that, because of the love they left here on earth, are allowed to let us know that they still exist.

Dr. Chopra is talking as a scientist and a physician about the "passing on." He grew up in India in a Hindu family, but he also went to a Catholic school. In his book *Life after Death*, he talks about both the Hindu and the Catholic approach to life after death. As a

Western physician, he is familiar with near-death experiences. The Hindu tradition is closer to Dr. Chopra than the Catholic tradition. He is familiar with science and is trying to explain the mysteries of life, death, and the afterlife, even if quantum science has failed to explain it. We all have a fear of inevitable death. Some people are so afraid of death that you can't even mention the word *death*. I think that using the information from NDE patients and the signs that our loved ones give us about their existence after death are safe ways to get at least a glimpse of what awaits us after we pass over. These experiences all point in one direction: namely that there is life after death and that we should better believe it while we can still prepare for it. We are making our own destiny in eternity right here on earth. After we cross over, we can't do anything anymore about our future life. We should better think about it now. It is known to us that we can't explain who God is. The resurrection of Jesus shows us that death is a transition. Jesus showed us that after we die, we would live again. This should be a big comfort to us.

Promise of Mercy

Dr. Williams F. Sullivan

The book *Promise of Mercy* was given to me at the University of Toronto St. Michael's College where I took a course on palliative care. William F. Sullivan, BSc, MD, CCFP, PhD (Phil.) wrote the book. Dr. Sullivan was the husband of a young woman with cancer. Her name was Connie Heng-Sullivan, whose experience of failure, loneliness, and illness became the fertile soil for new life in the Spirit. Despite being diagnosed with a terminal illness, Connie opened herself to God's love in a new way, married the love of her life, and became an example of hope and joy to both physicians and fellow patients (Sullivan 2002, 5). Connie showed us by her example of faith, hope, and love how to handle death with dignity (Sullivan 2002, "Introduction"). While writing about his wife, Dr. Sullivan mentions a dramatic conversion to the Catholic faith by Connie's father before his death.

Connie's father had always been a strong-willed atheist, and he liked to argue with Catholic missionaries. He had a very difficult time accepting his cancer; he became depressed and angry. Toward the end of his life, he refused to eat. During his stay in the Catholic hospital, he often asked to be wheeled into the chapel where he sat in darkness and silence. One morning, his wife found him sitting up in his hospital bed full of cheer. He wanted to eat. After he ate, he asked to see the Catholic chaplain right away. Dr. Sullivan writes that

Connie's father said that he had dreamed of a man in white, whom he identified as Jesus, who was trying to help him out of his wheelchair. Connie's father had experienced a joy that he had not felt since he had fallen ill. The chaplain baptized him the same day, and Connie's father died a few hours after that. Before Connie's father died, he asked his wife to become a Catholic and raise their children in the Catholic faith.

Dr. Sullivan writes in his book about what happened during the visit in the emergency department. He states that during his visit, when he was waiting with Connie in the emergency department, an elderly woman in the next bed kept shouting, "Nurse, there is a bird in the hospital." The nurse tried to reassure this woman that there was no bird in the department and told her not to disturb others. After that, Dr. Sullivan, John (Connie's brother), and Connie actually heard a bird chirping. Soon after that, the nurse checked on the woman next to Connie's bed and saw that she was dead. At that time, the birds' chirping stopped, and Connie's nausea vanished. From that time on, Connie did not have any nausea throughout her whole illness (Sullivan 2002, 41).

In his book *Promise of Mercy*, Dr. Sullivan writes about his wife's final phase of life in which she was completely immobilized after she began coughing up a large amount of blood and then lost consciousness. She was taken by ambulance to a local emergency department, where after several hours she regained consciousness. Dr. Sullivan writes in his book:

> While she was unconscious in the emergency department, we called Fr. Bob O'Brien to administer the Sacrament of the Sick. This was a powerful moment of prayer for all of us. Before Father Bob anointed Connie with the Oil of the Sick, he said to her, "You may not realize this, but you are a sign for us"…We discovered only later, when Connie had regained consciousness, that she not only

recalled the details of the Sacrament—what was said and by whom—but also a concurrent "dialogue" with Jesus and her predeceased relatives. (Sullivan 2002, 75)

Another thing that struck me while I was reading Dr. Sullivan's book about his wife, Connie, was the experience with the "wind." Dr. Sullivan describes it this way:

One of Connie's parting gifts to me personally was a mysterious encounter that we shared the day before she died. In the morning before I left for work, I paused to kiss her and felt a cool wind pass from her lips to my face, although it was not as though she had breathed on me. This "wind" seemed to fill my lungs and left me with a deep sense of peace and closeness, the likes of which I had not experienced before. (Sullivan 2002, 84)

Connie told Dr. Sullivan during her illness about her "windy experiences." Presence with her family occurred after her death at Christmastime. Connie's brother John lit a candle, which was to remember Connie and include her in the Christmas celebration. Dr. Sullivan mentions that in the midst of their gift exchange, Connie gave them her gift—a heart-shaped red drop of wax that had fallen from the candle that John had lit (Sullivan 2002, 90).

90 Minutes in Heaven: A True Story of Death and Life

DON PIPER

Don Piper writes that he was "standing in heaven after he flew throughout a long, dark tunnel without seeing any light. The only thing he recollected was the bridge and the rain. When he was standing in heaven, he experienced a brilliant light beyond human understanding" (Piper and Murphey 2004, 21).

Don Piper wanted to start a new congregation, and he wanted as much information as he could get about the process. He went to a conference where he could meet ministers with experience and knowledge about new church development. He wanted to know the hardships as well as the pitfalls to avoid. This conference was in January 1989, and Don died in a car accident following the convention on January 18, 1989. The author writes that paramedics reached the scene of the accident, and because they found no pulse, they declared Don Piper dead. A Baptist preacher came to the accident scene, and even though he knew that Don Piper was dead, he rushed to his lifeless body and prayed for him. The emergency medical technicians wanted him out of the scene of the accident, but he refused to stop praying. At least ninety minutes after the emergency medical technicians pronounced Don Piper dead, Don Piper came back to life.

RESEARCH INTO THE AFTERLIFE

In his book, Don describes his experiences in heaven. He remembered standing with other people in front of a brilliant, ornate gate. As the crowd of people rushed toward him, Don knew instantly that all of them had died during his lifetime. Everybody was smiling. The first person Don recognized was his grandfather. He called him by a nickname that his grandfather had always used. He embraced him, holding him tightly. The group showed their affection, greeting him warmly. Don Piper reported that "he had never felt more loved." He recognized a special friend from his childhood named Mike, who had encouraged Don to become a Christian. When Don was nineteen, Mike was killed in a car accident. Mike's death was very painful for Don, and when Don attended his funeral, he wondered if he would ever stop crying for Mike. Don didn't forget the pain and sense of loss from Mike's accident many years later, yet while his friend embraced him, Don's pain and grief vanished.

Many people came to welcome Don to heaven, and they were all very happy. Don's great-grandfather talked to him and embraced him. Many people that came to welcome Don to heaven hadn't known one another on earth, but they still seemed to know one another in heaven. They were all praising God. All the good people that had influenced his life in some way were waiting for him at the gates of heaven. Don Piper writes, "I could hardly grasp the vivid, dazzling colors. Every hue and tone surpassed anything I had ever seen" (Piper and Murphy 2004, 25). Don writes that he was not conscious of anything he had left behind. He had no regrets about leaving his family or possessions.

> Age expresses time passing, and there is no time there. All of the people I encountered were the same age, they had been the last time I had seen them—except that all the ravages of living on earth had vanished. Even though some of their features may not have been considered attractive on earth, in heaven every feature was perfect, beautiful and wonderful to gaze at. (Piper and Murphey 2004, 27)

While in heaven, Don was overwhelmed by the sound of music.

> My most vivid memory of heaven is what I heard…It was the most beautiful and pleasant sound I've ever heard, and it didn't stop. It was like a song that goes on forever. I felt awestruck, wanting only to listen. I didn't just hear music. It seemed as if I were part of the music—and it played in and through my body. I stood still and yet I felt embraced by the sounds. (Piper and Murphey 2004, 29–30)

Don also describes how he felt when he was in heaven:

> I saw colors I would never have believed existed. I've never, ever felt more alive than I did then. I was home; I was where I belonged. I wanted to be there more than I had ever wanted to be anywhere on earth. Time had slipped away, and I was simply present in heaven. All worries, anxieties, and concerns vanished. I had no needs, and I felt perfect…My words are too feeble to describe what took place. (Piper and Murphey 2004, 33)

Don described the gate made out of pearls, or according to him, pearl icing, similar to what the Bible refers to and what people saw after they died and what they described to their doctors after they were resuscitated back to life on earth. He paused just outside the gate, but he could see inside. He saw a city with paved streets. He describes it as streets paved with gold bricks, the same as what people that came back to life after they clinically died described to the doctors.

At the time of the accident, the truck went right over the top of Don's car. The truck smashed the car's ceiling and crushed his body. The EMTs pronounced Don Piper dead as soon as they arrived at the scene. They stated that he died instantly. Before the

EMT's were ready to move him, they checked his pulse once again. He was still dead.

A minister with his wife were among the people that were stuck with their car behind the accident. Dick and Anita Onerecker attended the same conference as Don. They decided to walk to the accident site. Dick asked the police officer if there was anyone he could pray for. He told him he was a minister. The police officer told him that the people were fine except the man in the red car, who was deceased. Later on, Dick told this story: "God spoke to me and said: 'You need to pray for the man in the red car'" (Piper and Murphey 2004, 42). When Dick asked the officer if he could pray for the man in the red car, the officer warned Dick that blood and glass were everywhere, and he said that he hadn't seen anything that bad before. Dick had to creep under the tarp which covered the car, and he put his hands on Don's shoulder. Dick felt compelled to pray for the man, even if he did not know who the man was. He was also singing. Dick prayed that the injured man could be delivered from his unseen injuries, especially brain and internal injuries, even if Dick knew that the man was dead.

While Dick was singing the hymn "What a Friend We Have in Jesus," Don began to sing with him. When Don regained his consciousness, he was aware of two things: he heard himself singing the hymn, and he was aware of someone clutching his hand. It was the first physical sensation that he experienced when he returned to earthly life. It was more than a year before Don understood the significance of that hand clasping his. He found out that Dick did not clasp his hand because Dick did not know where his hands were. When Don started to sing with Dick, Dick scrambled out of the smashed car and shouted, "The man is alive!" He was then shouting, "That man has come back to life!" (Piper and Murphey 2004, 45).

Dick had to try hard to get the remaining ambulance personnel to check on the man in the red car. Finally, the ambulance personnel raised the tarp, found Don's right arm, and felt his pulse. Then the action started, but they could not get Don out. They needed Jaws of Life to get Don out. Dick got back inside the car and continued to pray until the Jaws of Life arrived. Two hospitals refused to admit Don. Don had to go to Houston if he had any chance of survival.

Don started to have pain in every part of his body. The ambulance attendant said that he did all he could for his pain and that he couldn't let him go unconscious. Don finally arrived at the emergency room in Houston at Hermann Hospital. Six and a half hours had passed from the time of the accident. By the time Don reached the hospital in Houston, thousands of people were praying. Over the years, Don met many of those who asked God for his life. The prayers were effective; Don lived and is still alive. They finally sent Don to surgery, where he remained for eleven hours. When Don was conscious again, his pains were racing through his body. He hurt more than he thought was humanly possible (Piper and Murphey 2004, 51–53).

Don Piper writes that when Dick Onerecker came to see him at the hospital, he told Don that God told him to pray for no brain damage or any internal injuries. Doctors were amazed that Don had no head, internal, or thoracic injuries. The fact that the accident had not affected any of Don's internal organs defied all medical explanation. Don received thousands of cards and letters from people that believed in the power of prayer. Don Piper mentions that he lay in his bed with needles everywhere, unable to move, dependent on life-support apparatus. He had missing parts of bones in his left leg and his left forearm. He had to be put in traction. Don developed double pneumonia. The family was notified by the hospital that they did not think he would make it through the night. The doctors wanted to amputate Don's left leg because they thought it would save his life.

Don Piper writes that he did not want to live after he had been in heaven. He wanted to return to heaven. His friend David Gentiles drove nearly two hundred miles to see him. He told him that those who care for him would pray for him all night. The pneumonia was gone the next day. The mistake with the breathing tube that was inserted into his stomach instead of into his lungs was discovered. Don had to endure another twelve-hour surgery to save his left leg and received a bone-growth device.

The thought that God had a purpose in him staying alive by answering people's prayers kept Don going. After Don was discharged home from the hospital, he remained in bed for thirteen months and endured thirty-four surgeries. People prayed for Don. He knew that he would not die, but he still lived in depression. He wanted to be released from pain and go back to heaven. Don was thirty-eight years old, had three children and a wonderful wife. He was a man with a great future when the accident happened. After the accident, Don lived in humiliation. He had to have pain medication constantly, but no sleeping pill, pain shot, or additional morphine could put Don to sleep. Don needed a waterbed because of the bedsore on his back. The nurses had to clean the pinholes where the wires went into his skin and turn the screws of his left leg to cause the growing bone to replace the missing bone. This turn caused excruciating pain. Don could not sleep. He just passed out.

Even in his worst moment, Don did not forget that God had chosen to keep him alive (Piper and Murphey 2004, 73). Don was eventually able to do something doctors said he would never be able to do: he learned to walk again (Piper and Murphey 2004, 117). Don's depression lifted when he listened to the song "Praise the Lord." The whole song centers on praising God in spite of our circumstances. He also listened to the song "We Are the Reason." This song reminded Don that we are the reason Jesus Christ wept, suffered, and died on the cross. When he was listening to the songs, tears slid down his cheeks. He was reminded that Satan is a liar. He wants to steal our joy and replace it with hopelessness. Don was determined to get on with living the rest of his life no matter what.

Later on, Don was told that it was impossible to reach for his right hand. It was not Dick Onerecker whose hand gripped Don's hand and held it tight while he was praying for him under the tarp after the accident. The angel grasping his hand was God's way of sustaining Don and letting him know that he would not let go of him no matter how hard things become (Piper and Murphey 2004, 136). Don discovered one reason he could bring comfort to people who were facing death themselves or have suffered the loss of a loved one. He could give them every assurance that heaven is a place of unparalleled and indescribable joy. Without the slightest doubt, he knew heaven was real (Piper and Murphey 2004, pp. 129, 195).

Don was repeatedly thinking of the last night Jesus was with his disciples before his betrayal and crucifixion. Jesus begged them not to be troubled and to trust in him because he was going to his Father's house to prepare a place for them. Jesus told them that he would come back and take them with him so that they could be with him (Piper and Murphey 2004, 194–195). Don noticed that Jesus used the word *place*—a location. Don knows that it is a literal place and that heaven is real because he was there. Don has absolutely no fear of death. For him, there was nothing to fear, only joy to experience. He longs to return (Piper and Murphey 2004,195–196).

The Young Augustine

JOHN J. O'MEARA

While I was looking for books for my research, I came across a book about the young St. Augustine. St. Augustine was always a big interest to me. He was the son of St. Monica, for whom I have a huge amount of respect. She prayed for her son's conversion to Christianity. St. Augustine was born on the thirteenth of November AD 354. He was born in Africa at the time when the Romans conquered the land. Both husband and wife had worldly ambition for their son. His mother was a devout Christian, and his father was a pagan until just before his death. From Africa, St. Augustine went to Milan and Rome. He was honored with high office in Milan.

I decided to write about St. Augustine to show how God works in mysterious ways. The author writes that St. Augustine was wealthy. He was famous. He could have everything he wanted, but he preferred to follow Christ. His conversion took a long time, and it was very difficult. He joined the *Manichees*, a religious group/sect that rejected the Old Testament and "renounced most of the ordinary pleasures of life associated with eating, drinking and sexual expression" (McBrien, pp. 349–350). St. Augustine knew that he did not live according to Christian teachings. Many times, he was near to his conversion. He knew that he had to change, but he could not get rid of his lifestyle. This caused a controversy which St. Augustine could not solve. He was weeping bitterly in a garden where he was with a friend. He left the friend sitting on a bench and went to sit alone under a fig tree. At that time, he heard from a neighboring house a voice of a boy or girl chanting and repeating, "Take up and read, take up and read." St. Augustine interpreted it to be no other than a command from God to open the book and read the first chapter he should find. He stopped crying and returned to the place where his friend was sitting because he left a volume of the apostle there. He opened the book and in silence read that section on which his eyes fell. It was the writings of St. Paul (Romans 13:12–14).

> Not in rioting and drunkenness, not in chambering and wantonness, not in strife and envying: but put ye on the Lord Jesus Christ, and make not provision for the flesh, in concupiscence…No Further would I read; nor needed I: for instantly at the end of this sentence, by a light, as it were of serenity infused into my heart, all the darkness of doubt vanished away. (Confessions 8:28–29; O'Meara 1965, 179)

The conversion of Augustine, of his intellect which could not resist the truth, and of his will which could resist the good, was accomplished (O'Meara 1965, 179). It is customary to regard this episode as fully historical; that is to say that Augustine did cast himself down under a fig tree, weeping and asking God to deliver him from his bonds. What happened in the garden, the words that he read in the scriptures, changed St. Augustine's life. He was baptized at age thirty-three. He turned away from a sinful life; he gave it up completely. He became a Catholic Christian and was serving God as a bishop. His mother, St. Monica, who was praying for his conversion to Christianity, died shortly after his conversion. St. Augustine remained bishop for the rest of his life while living ascetically in community with his clergy until his death in AD 430 (McBrien, pp. 349–351).

At the Hour of Death or What They Saw at the Hour of Death

Dr. Karlis Osis and Dr. Erlandur Haraldsson

Dr. Karlis Osis and Dr. Erlandur Haraldsson looked into more than one thousand deaths or near-death experiences of patients on two continents: the United States and India. I will not talk too much about what I have read in this book because of the subject of apparitions that is very difficult to get into. I will just mention that the near-death experiences were similar in the Dr. Osis's scientific study as in the other books that I did the research on. Their reports support the theory of postmortem survival and acceptance of the afterlife hypothesis. Messages from the dead similar to mine from my late husband are also mentioned in this book, for example, clocks stopping, pictures falling, bells ringing, electric lights turning on, objects moved, and so on. For example, when Thomas A. Addison died, the clocks belonging to two of his associates stopped at the time of his death; his own grandfather clock stopped only a few minutes later (Osis and Haraldsson 1977, 44). In my book, I wanted to concentrate on the research dealing with life after death as clinical death survivors explain it. The knowledge about life after death brings me peace of mind that my husband is alive in a different dimension and that he let me know about his existence. This knowledge is very comforting to me.

Jung on Death and Immortality

JENNY YATES

*D*r. Carl Gustav Jung lived from 1875 to 1961. He was a pioneer in psychoanalysis. One of Jung's main interest in the area of psychology, spirituality, and personal growth was immortality. He made every effort to strengthen the belief in immortality, especially with older patients, when such questions came close. He once wrote that death is psychologically important and, like it, is an integral part of life. He said that seen in correct psychological perspectives, death is not an end but a goal (Yates 1999, 3).

The author writes that Jung started to be interested in life after death after his father's death. He had a dream in which his father appeared to him and told him that he would be coming home. "In his writings, Jung explains how the soul or spirit descends into the unconscious or the land of the dead and activates the contents, like a medium, giving those who are dead a chance to manifest" (Yates 1999, 4). The author writes that in January 1944, Jung himself had a near-death experience following a heart attack. The description suggests a transient cardiac arrest. In *Memories, Dreams, Reflections*, Jung describe his out-of-body experience and his vision of the globe with its alchemical silver earth and reddish-gold hue. Jung's near-death experience is in accord with phenomena recently discussed by doctors who have resuscitated patients after they have died a clinical death (Yates 1999, 6). Because of the experience when his wife,

Emma, died in 1955, he believed in a strong link between husband and wife in death. In his writings before, he spoke of the inner marriage that forms a window to eternity (Yates 1999, 8).

The author writes that in his work, Jung suggested that dreams are a clue to understanding life after death. According to Jung, life is an energy process and is therefore directed toward a goal. Jung talks about death as a goal, but most people consider death as the end and don't think about the continuation of life. I hope that after reading my book, those people will think about death differently. The author mentions that people can also be comforted by the notion that, by dying, a transformation of a mortal into an immortal being, a corporeal into a spiritual being, takes place: a transformation of a human being into a divine being.

> Well-known prototypes of this change are the transfiguration and ascension of Christ and the assumption of the Mother of God into heaven after her death, together with her body…Christ is the perfect example of the hidden immortal within the mortal man. All of us are immortal, but we don't want to believe it. God gave us a free will and with this free will, we can do whatever we want and believe whatever we want. (Yates 1999, 38)

In a letter dated January 10, 1939, Jung responded to Pastor Fritz Pfafflin's inquiries about a conversation the pastor had with his brother at the time of his brother's death, although a continent separated them. Jung wrote:

> It is very probable that only what we call consciousness is contained in space and time, and that the rest of the psyche, the unconscious, exists in a state of relative spacelessness and timelessness. For the psyche this means

a relative eternity and relative non-separation from other psyches, or an oneness with them. (Yates 1999, 6)

According to Jung, the timeless and spaceless relativity allows the "continual presence of the dead and their influence on our dream life...After a few months this ceases; the danger of lingering too long can lead to dissociation" (Yates 1999, 6).

I once had a dream myself in which I was walking beside a man whom I thought was my husband, but I was not sure of it. I was overcome by an indescribable peace and happiness, which ended when the man turned to me and then was standing in front of me. The man was my husband. With this, the dream ended. I still remember the dream, but I can't imagine the incredible happiness anymore.

According to Jung, death is the hardest thing from the outside as long as we are outside of it; but inside death, you feel a sense of completeness, peace, and fulfillment, and you don't want to return to life. Jung described how after the first month of his vision, he suffered from depression because he felt that he was recovering. He didn't want to leave and return to the narrow, almost mechanical life.

Jung once wrote that death is brutal and that there is no sense pretending otherwise. It is brutal not only as a physical event but far more brutal psychically. From another point of view, however, Jung writes that death appears as a joyful event because the soul achieves wholeness. According to Jung, if people knew that what truly matters is the infinite, people would stop fixing their interest upon all kinds of goals which are not of real importance. He writes that people demand recognition for qualities like our talent and our beauty. He writes that concentrating on false possessions results in envy and jealousy, which makes people less satisfied with their lives. Jung writes that if people would understand that in this life, we already have a link with the infinite, our desires and attitudes would change. Jung wrote to an anonymous person that what happens after death is so unspeakably glorious that our imagination and our feelings do not suffice to form even an approximate conception of it (Yates 1999, 160).

In another anonymous letter, Jung writes that the psyche is capable of telepathic and precognitive perceptions. To that extent, it exists in a continuum outside time and space. We may therefore expect postmortem phenomena to occur, which must be regarded as authentic.

> The comparative rarity of such phenomena suggests at all events that the forms of existence inside and outside time are so sharply divided that crossing this boundary presents the greatest difficulties. But this does not exclude the possibility that there is an existence outside time which runs parallel with existence inside time. (Yates 1999, 161)

Jung regards postmortem phenomena that are occurring as authentic, which I am trying to prove. By writing this book about the immortality and about the existence of a soul, I am trying to prove that the signs that my husband gave us after his death were done through his immortal spirit.

Into the Light

DR. JOHN LERMA

In his book *Into the Light*, Dr. John Lerma shares his research information for children and adults in sixteen stories of predeath experiences of visions of divine beings. I have heard about these visions also in other books where other doctors wrote about near-death experiences and reported these visions. He shares with the reader what the dying patients told him. They told Dr. Lerma that their suffering is part of their learning experience. A blind cancer patient, a very special nine-year-old boy, reported that he could see angels in his room. He told Dr. Lerma that the angels took him to beautiful places. When Dr. Lerma asked him what heaven is like, he said that it is like earth, but it is perfect. Dr. Lerma told a mother of a two-year-old boy about it. The mother wanted her little Jacob to be with God and the angels when he died. She was Jewish, and according to her religion, her son was supposed to go to a place called She'ol and wait for their Messiah to resurrect him. The mother was praying for a sign to know that her child was in heaven. The child had no strength in his muscles for several months. When he was dying, Dr. Lerma was on his bed and witnessed what had happened:

> Jacob opened his eyes, smiled really big, and raised his arms as if he was reaching for someone above him. Dr. Lerma was stunned. It was impossible for the child to rally

that kind of muscle strength. Jacob died with a smile on his face. Jacob's brother, Michael, a 4-year-old boy wanted to sit next to his mother, but sat on the other side of the bed. His mother wanted to know why he moved to the other side of the bed. He told her that there was an angel sitting next to her so he could not sit there. Later on, after Michael went into the hallway, he came back crying. He said that angels are playing with Jacob and told him that Jacob's body is just a shell.

One of the accounts given to Dr. John Lerma was a conversation with a well-respected and well-loved retired Catholic priest, a renowned theologian. He was diagnosed with head, neck, and lung cancer. Father Mike was missing one eye, and the remaining eye had severe cataract. Father Mike did not want any pain medication. He wanted to feel his pain in its most raw form. This was a tremendous conflict for Dr. Lerma. Father Mike believed in the positive effects of pain on people. He allowed Dr. Lerma to take notes while he was talking to him about what the pain was teaching him. Father Mike said that watching the negative aspects of world and local news affects our souls in a dark way, and puts us in a position to develop fear and judgment of others, without even trying. This compounds the negativity in our souls and this truly hurts God. The angels he spoke with talked about working on many projects to improve optimism in the world. One of those was to increase the number of workers in the entertainment and news that are God-loving. (Lerma 2007, 121)

Father Mike said that people can address the issues of war, famine, and diseases through peace, love, and technology. He said that technology will have to integrate with spirituality. He did not receive any pain medication even if he was in distress. He remained at peace with a large smile. On the day Father Mike died, Dr. Lerma was at his clinic across the street. There was a storm while Dr. Lerma received a page that Father Mike had passed and that he needed to come immediately. When he arrived, the lights at the hospice floor were flickering on and off. Dr. Lerma writes in his book that every time the lights turned on and off, little feathers fell from the ceiling as if they were snowflakes. When they fell in the hands of nurses, they disappeared. Father Mike's call light was also going off and on, and his door was now open, which had been closed before. Bright light was shining from his room. The light was radiating from Father Mike's body or bed. The light circled the bed about three times and then soared out of the closed window. The lights came back on. It stopped raining, and all the feathers disappeared. The people that were present had goose bumps.

When Father Mike died, he had a smile on his face, and the eye that had the cataract seemed to have cleared. People that were present during these events thought that the lights had something to do with the storm, but they were not able to explain the feathers. The dean knew that Father Mike collected feathers all his life. When he went to Father Mike's office, he noticed that all the feathers were gone.

Dr. Lerma writes that he and Father Mike had many discussions. Father Mike said that we have to be wise in order to survive. Father Mike agreed with Einstein, who said that as a human race, we are in danger of becoming extinct because the financially and physically strong have been allowed to impose their will on others.

Dr. Lerma hopes that we will take Father Mike's advice and cultivate spirituality and technology together. Another interesting story Dr. Lerma talks about in his book is about a phone call that he and also a son of a deceased woman received just after that person died. While dying, the woman said to Dr. Lerma that she was worried about her son. Her son never married and had nobody to comfort him. He wanted to know that his mother made it to heaven. Dr. Lerma writes in his book that the mother did not want her son to be with her when she was dying. It happened that her son had a car problem and could not come in the morning the day she was dying. When Dr. Lerma was leaving the room where the patient was dying, he turned and saw a whisk of white smoke rise from her opened mouth. He pronounced her time of death. The nurse tried several times to reach her son to notify him that his mother died, but the telephone line was repeatedly busy.

A couple of hours after her death, Dr. Lerma was at the nurses' station, and the phone rang. The caller identification showed the number of the room where this woman had just died a couple of hours earlier. The nurse picked the phone and looked confused. She handed the phone to Dr. Lerma. Dr. Lerma heard a lot of static and a distant voice saying, "Tell my son I'm okay. Tell my son I'm okay." Dr. Lerma and the nurse went into that room where the woman died. Dr. Lerma checked her and found her quite cold and dead. About half an hour later, her son arrived. Dr. Lerma told him that his mother had passed. Dr. Lerma shared his mother's words. The son told Dr. Lerma that when she'd phoned him an hour ago, he thought she was alive and that they just had a bad connection. There was a lot of static, but she kept saying, "Isaac, I am okay. I love you. Don't worry about me. I am okay." He thought that she was calling from the hospital, so he kept trying to phone Dr. Lerma to see what was going on with her. Dr. Lerma said that he believes that love is the strongest force in the universe (Lerma 2007, 173).

The last case that I want to present to the reader from Dr. Lerma's book *Into the Light* is of Dr. Jean Pierre. He was a sixty-seven-year-old anthropological pathologist and agnostic who was dying of multiple myeloma. This highly intelligent and stoic individual had two weeks before his death. Dr. Lerma states that despite his pain, Dr. Jean Pierre was filled with inner joy. He described the spiritual entity he called "Michael" as a cosmic being.

Dr. Jean Pierre said that because he did not know if God existed, Michael was sent to help him attain the yearning to move toward God. Dr. Jean Pierre talked to Dr. Lerma about Michael. He said that Michael discussed the importance of spirituality and science with regard to space travel. He said that it may be perfected by science in the near future, resulting in interstellar and intergalactic travel through the use of advanced propulsion systems, amplified gravity, antimatter, and even wormholes. He gave details of meeting other peaceful souls not only in our galaxy but in the far reaches of the universe. He emphasized that this accomplishment could only be realized if scientists would believe in God. He said that through spirituality comes peace and love. Without this, humans would infect the rest of creation with hatred, pride, and arrogance (Lerma 2007, 213–215).

Michael informed Dr. Jean Pierre about God's creation starting with the big bang to the first *Homo sapiens*. Michael said that God gave us a free will and is deeply saddened by man destroying the environment and one another. "He said that the body was engineered to house our soul, to give us the necessary experiences, knowledge, and wisdom seek and return to God in the hereafter. That is why securing the planet's existence is crucial" (Lerma 2007, 215–218).

Dr. Jean Pierre was a scientist, and he understood for the first time that science without God was virtually limited and that science with God was unlimited. Dr. Jean Pierre explains that the majority of people are God-loving, and they will evolve in technology, medicine, and spirituality. Michael told Dr. Jean Pierre that God did not want robots to share in his kingdom. He explained that God wanted human beings to love him for him as he loved us for us (Lerma 2007, 220).

Dr. Jean Pierre told Dr. Lerma never to forget that energy has just changed form and never dies. He said that the same holds true for our soul, which will exist for eternity and hopefully will not be separated from our loving Creator. He said that, after all, it is all about free will. He said that hell is definitely a self-separation from God as God never wants to separate from us. He also said that anything is possible with God. He mentions that all we have to do is believe (Lerma 2007, 222).

Dr. Lerma mentions in his book that Einstein also explained through the theory of relativity that energy is neither created nor destroyed; it only changes form. The idea of postmortem survival and pre death visions did not appear suddenly. They have been mentioned by different scientists in different books, several of which I have mentioned in my bibliography and also by well-known people like Abraham Lincoln. President Lincoln reported that in his dream, he heard some subdued sobs as if a number of people were weeping. He dreamed that he went from room to room until he arrived at the East Room, which he entered. There he saw a catafalque on which rested a corpse. He asked who died in the White House, and the soldier replied, "The president…he was killed by an assassin." President Lincoln awoke from his dream and could not sleep anymore. At the end of his book, Dr. Lerma mentions that several pilot studies about the afterlife were supportive of the afterlife hypothesis.

Dr. Lerma writes that despite our advancements in science and medicine, death and life after death remains a mystery.

Heaven Is for Real

TODD BURPO WITH LYNN VINCENT

Colton Burpo was almost four years old when he had a near-death experience. During his emergency appendectomy for a burst appendix, Colton went through an experience that he describes as a trip to heaven and back. First, Colton described what his parents were doing in another part of the hospital during his operation. He told his father that he saw him praying and his mommy talking on the phone. Colton said that he went up out of his body and was looking down and could see the doctor working on his body. That was an experience consistent with an out-of-body experience. Sometimes people have an out-of-body experience and a near-death experience at the same time. Colton further told his parents that he was in heaven, that he saw Jesus, the angels, his sister, John the Baptist, and Pop. Pop was Colton's paternal great-grandfather. Colton never met him because Pop was dead for some time. Colton said that nobody was old in heaven. When asked what Colton wants people to know from his story, Colton replied that he wants people to know that heaven is for real and that God really, really loves us.

Colton told his father that when he was in heaven, there were lots of colors and that Jesus has red markers, by which he meant red scars from the crucifixion. He also said that Jesus had a part of purple clothes on top of white or a sash, but Colton had not known the word *sash* yet. When Colton spoke to his father, his father realized that Colton was an eyewitness. Colton said that there were lots of kids in heaven. He talked to his father about what he saw in heaven and that he had to do homework. It seemed like a lot of time that Colton spent in heaven, but when his father asked how long he was there, Colton said that he was in heaven for three minutes. The Bible says that with the Lord "a day is like a thousand years, and a thousand years are like a day" (Burpo 2010, 78). It looks like there is not the same time in heaven as on earth. The medical staff never gave any report to Colton's parents saying that Colton had ever been clinically dead.

Todd Burpo was wondering how Colton could come to heaven if he had not died. As a pastor, Todd remembered that the Bible talks in several places about people who had seen heaven without dying. He remembered that John the apostle described heaven in great detail in the book of Revelation. The author mentions that the apostle Paul wrote to the church at Corinth about a Christian whom he knew personally who was taken to heaven and did not die. Colton told his father that Jesus said that he had to go back because he was answering his father's prayer. As a matter of fact, Todd, Colton's father, yelled at God, chastised him, and questioned his wisdom and his faithfulness during his prayer. His father wondered why God would answer a prayer like that.

Colton told his father that he met Pop. Pop was Todd's mother's dad. Colton said that Pop told him that Todd and Pop had a lot of fun together when Todd visited him. Todd was about six years old when his grandfather died in a car accident. Colton told his grandma about her dad. Pop had recognized his great-grandson even though Colton was born decades after Pop died. That got Colton's grandmother wondering whether those who have gone ahead of us know what's happening on earth.

The author writes that Colton told his parents that he saw his other sister in heaven. His parents never told Colton that his mother had a miscarriage when the baby was only tiny. He said that the baby was a girl and that she ran up to him and wouldn't stop hugging him in heaven. He told his parents that she did not have a name because her parents did not give her a name yet. He told his father that he saw God the Father sitting on the big chair, which his father explained to Colton is called the throne. Colton said that Jesus's chair is right next to his Dad's. He pointed to the right side of Todd. He also said that Angel Gabriel is on the other side of God's throne. Colton said that he himself was sitting with God the Holy Spirit on a little chair.

When Todd asked what the Holy Spirit looked like, Colton said that he was kind of blue. He said that there was always light in heaven. When the parents showed Colton the picture of Pop in which Pop was sixty-one years old and wearing glasses, he did not recognize him, but he recognized him from the picture in which Pop was twenty-nine years old. A lot of Catholics asked if Colton saw Mary, the mother of Jesus. The answer was that he saw Mary kneeling before the throne of God and, at other times, standing beside Jesus. In today's time, when people question the existence of God, Pastor Todd Burpo was always comfortable talking about his faith, but now he also talks about what happened to his son.

Colton said, "Everybody in heaven has wings. Everyone except Jesus." "Jesus just went up and down like in an elevator." "All the people have a light above their head" (Burpo 2010, 72–73). He also said that "the flowers and trees in heaven were beautiful and there were animals of every kind" (Burpo 2010, 105).

WHY SHOULD WE BELIEVE IN LIFE AFTER DEATH?

*B*ecause to talk about death is "taboo" in our society, people may not get a proper understanding of what I am talking about when I describe my experiences with the signs that my husband gave me after his death. Reading about it, people may not understand the real meaning behind it, even if they find the significance of it. There is no scientific explanation of what has happened to me. I opened the Bible exactly on the page that I wanted to find, and I did not know the content of the Bible before. How can I explain that? It is not easy to write a book of this calibre in such a way that people can understand it immediately. When I opened the Bible on the page that I wanted to find, I was startled. I started to cry. I phoned my friend and told her what happened. She said, "I think it was your husband who opened the Bible for you." I knew that it was my husband who did it; I just needed to hear it from other people. My husband was with me in the house, but I could not see him. I told this to a doctor who knew my husband. I asked him if he thought it was coincidence. He said, "No, it was your husband."

How can science explain why the light switched off in the bathroom at the time when I wanted to do it? The lights in the other rooms were working, and it was not the breaker. The light was working again when I came back from my walk. Nobody was in the cottage when I was away. I know that atheists and agnostics will try to disprove what I am writing about, but they won't be able to explain it. A few months after my husband's death, I heard my husband's command: "Live." No dream preceded it. Where did this command come from? I talked to people about it, and some of them told me that they had a real conversation with their dead loved ones, or they heard them say more than one word. They would not lie to me.

A university professor heard her father calling her name for four years. Why would she tell me that if it would not be true? She did not have to tell me about it. I know that people who had this kind of experiences will believe me, but I would like other people to believe me too. Would people believe me that I heard the doorknob turning on my bedroom door in the cottage one week after my husband died? I know that it was my husband who did it. Would people believe me that I heard footsteps on the balcony behind my window in the cottage during the night? It did not scare me. I knew that the footsteps were not from a person because they were very regular, and I heard those footsteps for a while on the roof too. They were close to the end of the roof on the same side as the balcony. I was not dreaming; I was sitting on my bed. I was alone in the cottage. Those footsteps were going on and on. Why did it not scare me?

Finally, I felt tired. I lay on my bed, and I fell asleep immediately. Why did I hear those steps also on the roof? To make sure that I know that those steps were not from a person but by a divine force? There are many questions that nobody can answer for me. I am sure that people who will read about my experiences will have questions too, but they can at least know about the signs that people get over the death of their loved ones. Many people have heard footsteps on the floor after the death of people whom they loved to let them know about their existence, but nobody writes about it. Those people can confirm what I am writing about.

WHY SHOULD WE BELIEVE IN LIFE AFTER DEATH?

What happened to the rosary that disappeared from my husband's car and came back after two days? This is the most incredible of all signs I received from my husband. My husband hung the white plastic rosary on the rear-view mirror about two years before his death. Some of his patients that I talked to remembered the rosary hanging on that mirror. The patients knew my husband's car. It was parked in front of his office. My husband's car was a leased car. At the end of the lease, the Ford dealership sent one of their representatives to check the car if it was in a good condition to be brought back to the company. When the representative came, he checked the car and gave the key back to me. The rosary was hanging on the mirror when he came to inspect the car. The next day, I noticed that there was no rosary. I got alarmed. I thought that I was getting Alzheimer's disease because I did not remember that I removed the rosary. I told this to my older son, and he said that it might be inside the house. I looked for it twice inside the house, but I did not find it. I checked the car twice, but no rosary.

It was already said before that I found the rosary two days later in the corner of the mat. When I found the rosary, I was angry. I put the rosary inside my pocket, and when I came home from my son's house, I threw the rosary beside my phone, and I said, "You made me believe that I am getting Alzheimer's disease." I think that I sensed my husband's presence beside me. After I said that, I realized that I was alone, and I started to cry and asked my husband for forgiveness in my mind. I realized that the rosary was handled. The rosary was removed from the car and put back inside the car by my husband. There is no other explanation. St. Thomas Aquinas said in his *Summa Theologica* that the soul has a body and can move. It is unbelievable, I know. I wish I could find some trustworthy literature about this kind of phenomenon, but people just don't write about the signs that they get from their dead loved ones. It is "taboo." Dr. Wilder Penfield also said before his death that the soul has energy. If it has energy, then it can move!

The incident with the maple trees that I describe in this book can't be explained scientifically either. My sons were cutting the little maple trees that grew in my raspberry patch one late Sunday afternoon when the sun went down. My younger son called on me, "Mom, why do you have lights on in the sunroom? You are wasting electricity!" I said that I did not put the light on. I asked my daughter and my daughter-in-law if they put the light on, and they said that they did not. I switched off the light. After everybody was gone, I noticed that the light was on again. I switched it off for the second time. I was wondering what was going on. The next day, I phoned some electric companies and asked if it was possible for the light to come on by itself. All of them told me that it was not possible.

A few days later, a patient came to pick up his medical file. He was an electrician. I asked him too if the light could switch on by itself. He said that it could happen only if the wires had expended by extensive heat and touched each other. This was not the case. The only explanation for me was that the light was put on by the soul of my husband for the first time to show all of us that he was with us, and the second time to show me that it was he who put it on. I have heard from other people that they too had experienced flickering of the light after the death of a loved one. It is not possible to explain these events scientifically. We can only hope that one day we will be able to gain more knowledge about the soul and what it can do here on earth.

I think that God doesn't want us to know everything. He gives us some hints about himself, but he doesn't disclose himself fully because he showed us enough through his Son and his Son's resurrection. His Son's resurrection is documented in Christian and Jewish writings. The proof of Jesus's suffering and death is shown to us from the Shroud of Turin, which was finally proved to be authentic. The fourteen-foot relic is evidence of Jesus's rising from death. It is the only record of how he looked like. It is the most venerated relic for us. It is God's story presented to us human beings.

WHY SHOULD WE BELIEVE IN LIFE AFTER DEATH?

In 1988, the Vatican gave a piece of the shroud for carbon testing to be done in three different places: London, Zurich, and Arizona. The conclusion of the testing was that the shroud is a clever thirteenth-century forgery. Later on, a sudarium (a piece of cloth with stains of blood on it) showing Jesus's face was found. This piece of cloth was put on Jesus's face when Joseph of Arimathaea and Nicodemus were taking Jesus down from the cross. It was taken away when the body of Jesus was wrapped in linen cloths, following the Jewish burial custom. When Jesus's body was wrapped in linen cloths and put into the tomb, the piece of cloth from his head was put beside him. This piece of cloth was also tested after it was found, and the result was that it is seven hundred years older than the previously tested piece of shroud. This is the time when Jesus was crucified.

Scientists found out now that the Shroud of Turin contains human blood and not red paint as it was believed in 1988. Scientists also found out that Jesus was crucified from the wrist, not from the hand, as it was believed before. The shroud also shows the place where Jesus was pierced. It shows the blood and water that came out of that place. The comparison of the places of injury on the face showed the same places on the Shroud of Turin and the same places on the piece of cloth with Jesus's face on it. On the account of these findings, the Shroud of Turin was changed from a clever forgery to an authentic piece of evidence. It is believed now that it was the body of Jesus that was wrapped in the shroud.

According to Christian and Jewish writings, the tomb was found empty on the third day after the crucifixion. The Shroud of Turin is scientific evidence that Jesus lived, was crucified, died, and was risen. These findings should satisfy the atheists and the agnostics. Jesus's resurrection is the best record of life after death. After his resurrection, Jesus appeared to about five hundred people here on earth. There are written records about that in the Bible. People that were writing about it saw Jesus during that time, and they died for Jesus. How much more proof of afterlife do we need?

Our departed loved ones are showing us that they live on, but we don't believe them. We want science to explain it to us, but science can't explain it.

Another reason why we don't want to believe in life after death is that we believe in the theory of evolution the way Darwin portrayed it. Darwin wanted us to believe that life on earth started without God. The existence of God and the possibility of an afterlife lie outside the scientific method. The search for God is universal. If people are supposed to believe in life after death, they first have to believe in God. There is a proposition that the theory of evolution is flawed. Life is very complex. One hundred and fifty years ago, the living cell was thought to be something that has evolved, but since that time, there have been many new discoveries in science. Scientists now know that the cell is too complex and could not have just happened. The cell had to have been designed. Evolutionary biologists would have to explain in detail how the biochemical systems originated all on their own if they want us to believe them. According to astronomers, there is not enough time and resources available throughout the universe's history to generate life in its simplest form. Evolutionary biologists would have to demonstrate using the available time and resources at their disposal that life had an evolutionary origin for us to believe them.

I had to write about all that because if people will not believe in God, they can't believe in life after death. I want people to believe in life after death, and therefore, I am also talking about God, even if it is very difficult for me to explain him. People should try to find God through nature. I personally admire nature. I love flowers and birds. I admire the flowers for their beauty and nice smell and the birds for their songs and freedom to go to different places fast. They also look beautiful. People who died a clinical death reported seeing more beautiful, bigger, and more colorful flowers in the place where they have been during their clinical death. There is nothing for us to fear if we will stay good people. There is a beautiful place prepared for us in eternity. There is a lot of evidence now that life must have been created. Life is of a supernatural origin; it is the work of an intelligent Designer. God was revealed to us in the Scriptures. He wants us to know about him.

The Epilogue

Jesus told us many times that there is life after death, but we could never understand it. Jesus knew that we don't understand that he is both divine and human. He told Peter that Peter was a happy man because he knew that Jesus was Christ, the Son of the living God. He said, "Because it was not flesh and blood that revealed this to you, but my Father in heaven" (Matthew 16:17–18). Jesus wanted us to know that we will live again after we die. He knew that it would be difficult for us to understand it.

It is difficult to believe in life after death, even if Jesus told us two thousand years ago about it. We don't believe him even if he promised to build a place for us. How many people in history really understood Jesus's words? For two thousand years after Jesus's death, people are still searching if there is life after death. Some people that died gave us signs that they were living again. Do we believe that it is true? We are trying through science to disprove it. But quantum science can't disprove it. Quantum science disappointed scientists, and therefore, they are putting together a new science. If a light switched off by itself, how can we explain it? If I open a Bible on exactly the same place which I wanted to find, and I did not know the contents of the Bible before, how can I explain that? If a light comes on two times in a row by itself, how can I explain that? Many things have happened to people after a loved one died that are against the rules of science and are not explainable. How about the people that died a clinical death and came back to life and told us what they had seen? Do we believe them? Their brains did not function at the time of their death, so how did they see what they had seen? What is a soul or spirit or mind? Every human being struggles with it. Everybody is afraid of death. It troubles us every day. Jesus said that we should not let our hearts be troubled about it. Do we listen to him?

How do we learn about life after death if we have no way to find out, only through what God reveals to us, which we don't take seriously? To write this book was very painful for me. I always believed that all the signs that were given to me were from my husband, but my children tried to find some logical explanation for it. After I told my relatives about the signs, I knew that they did not believe that they were from my husband, and some of them thought that I had gone insane. Who helped me most in my time of despair were my husband's patients. Almost everybody I talked to knew someone to whom similar things had happened. Some of them told me about their own experiences. I will be forever thankful to all the people who shared their stories with me. The idea of the existence of the spirit was in my mind constantly, but I could not understand it.

After the two words *quantum mechanics* formed in my mind, I felt like forgetting the whole book, but I was not supposed to do that. The book by John Polkinghorne helped me understand that as much as quantum science can't explain what we need to have explained, theology can't explain many things either. I will be forever indebted to John Polkinghorne for explaining the problems with quantum science, as well as problems with the theology in his book *Quantum Physics and Theology: An Unexpected Kinship*. I understood that I couldn't write this book without suffering and without an honest study. After having read all those thirty-three books, I realized that the connection between life and death is love. Because of the love I shared with my husband, which did not die but still continues after his death, I was able to hear and receive signs from him so that I would be informed that he still exists. Love lives forever.

Many people received signs from people that loved them after those people died; I am not the only one. Those people will be happy that I did research about the afterlife, and they will look forward to seeing their loved ones again. I have learned that if there is love between people, then after the transition from this life to another existence, the person who made the transition may be allowed to let their loved ones know about their existence. I had to do research on life after death. I did it! What a relief to find out that what I suspected was true. My husband is living in eternity, and I will see him again! It took me a lot of searching, reading, and writing to find the truth. Nobody can tell me now that I am insane because there is evidence that there is life after death. I am giving the reader the names of those who did scientific research together with the titles of the books they had written on the evidence of the afterlife.

I could never imagine life without my husband. He was a part of me, and he still is. When I was with my husband, I did not care about my age. I felt young. I felt like I was the same age as when we met. What I had learned in those books that I researched was that the soul doesn't get old. According to research, it takes an average widow many years after her spouse's death to regain her level of life satisfaction. What I am not able to understand is the fact that while the signs from my husband were happening, I was never frightened, and I was always confident that the signs were from him. I had to do the research to understand it. I think that we all should try to learn more, to understand more. We all have questions. We all want to know who we are. Why are we here on earth? Why can't we live in peace? Why are we constantly longing for something that we can't explain? Why can't we be happy? I think that we all should try to educate ourselves, to learn more about life. We should learn that this life is not the only one there is, that there is another everlasting life awaiting us.

Metaphysics can teach us about it. What I learned from all the books that I had read is that God loves all of us, that we all can come to him. I have also learned that there is an evil force that doesn't want to be discovered. People of goodwill should conquer this evil force together. If we are scared to talk about evil, there will be more evil. We should not let the minds of children be corrupted by evil. Half of marriages are ending in divorce. Why? The reason is because people are influenced by evil. What happened to love? I believe that prayer to God should not be taken out of schools. Sometimes it is the only prayer children will hear if prayer is not said in the family. How else should children hear that there is God, whom they will meet one day?

Nobody ever found out who created the earth and all the living things in it. God sent his Son to tell us about him. Nobody had ever seen God, but we have seen his Son, Jesus. There are many things that we can't see, but they exist. How about the atom? We can't see atoms, but they exist. We don't believe in spirits because we can't see them. People who died clinically and were resuscitated back to life saw them and communicated with them. They can also let us know here on earth that they exist. Some people don't believe in the afterlife, but it is written in the Bible. Some people don't believe in what is written in the Bible, and they say that the New Testament was written too long after Jesus died. Yes, but the New Testament was circulating among Christians in short versions after Jesus died and was written by the same people that lived with Jesus. It was put in a book form later on. These people saw Jesus, listened to him, and knew him well. They saw Jesus and talked to Jesus even after his resurrection for forty days. During those forty days, they touched him and ate with him. Should we think that those people made it all up? They did not need to do that; they had nothing to gain from it. On the contrary, they have been persecuted, and some of them died for their beliefs. Would they not rather live? They must have seen something for which they would rather die than deny! God wants us to know him. Even this book is a testimony that he exists.

I have done research about life after death that is based on testimonies of people that died a clinical death. These testimonies are documented all over the world. Can sceptics disprove the doctors who did the scientific investigations about life after death? Jesus's resurrection is a fact. It has been documented. His resurrection is the most powerful testimony of life after death. We should remind ourselves about his death and resurrection as much as possible. Why do some Christians think that it is wrong to have the cross or the cross with the suffering Jesus on it in the house or in the church? I could never understand that. Some Christians also think that it is wrong to have a statue of the mother of Jesus in the house or in the church. They call it an idol. It is not an idol. People don't pray to the statue or the picture; they pray to the one whom they are reminding them of. Christians are against other Christians just because of that. There is just one God, and people should not be against one another just because they belong to a different religion. After my husband died, a Hindu family who wanted me to live in their house with them until my mourning for my husband would improve approached me. What an act of love from a non-Christian! I will never forget about that.

What I have learned from all the books that I have read and from what people who have died clinically have reported is that life-after-death experiences from all over the world are similar, regardless of religion. All the people were treated equally when they died clinically. So is the being of light they reported as a supernatural according to their religion and beliefs. I think that we can conclude that we are all God's beings, no matter what our religious beliefs are. Some people told me that Jesus said, "Nobody can come to the Father, only through me." Those people don't know what he meant. People who reported what they saw during their clinical death said that they went to a place of incredible beauty, but it was not yet heaven; it looked like a gathering place. They were aware that there was heaven just beside that place, but they were sent back to earth to finish their earthly journey. Maybe the being of light is Jesus, who decides who will go to heaven and can see God the Father. This way, we can understand why Jesus said, "Nobody will come to the Father, only through me." He did not say that you have to be a Christian to be able to see his Father. Nobody from those people who died and were resuscitated back to life said that they have seen God the Father. They have seen a being of light.

By reading all the different books in order to understand the unexplainable, I learned that God created physical laws for the universe and moral laws for human beings. If we human beings will not live according to those moral laws, we will encounter bad consequences. The same will happen if we try to change the laws of nature. God created nature according to his laws. He has a plan. If we try to work against his law and his plan, we will create problems for all of us. God gave us the earth for nourishment. We should not destroy it.

The more I talk to people, the more I can see how unhappy they are. We are unhappy because we don't want to understand what God is showing us. God shows us that he exists by what he created. We want science to explain to us what we don't understand, but science can't explain it. What will we do? If we believe in the theory of evolution, where did this longing for the loving presence of God come from? God created us for himself, but he doesn't want puppets that will do what he wants them to do. He gave us free will. He wants people that will recognize him and live according to his laws and love him. As a medical secretary, I saw problems that people caused to themselves and to other people when they did not live according to God's commandments. God's commandments are here to stay.

Once we start to think about the design and the purpose of the Creator of the universe, we start to think of whom this splendour was created for, we start to think about the afterlife. Just watch a movie about the universe. You will start to think more about God. God is the Creator of the universe, and he has the plan. Did Darwin really think that all the creation came about from nothing and without a purpose? Why do we experience this longing for eternal life? Does Darwin's theory of evolution talk about it? I know that it is difficult to understand what is really happening to us. I am the same as anybody else, but I am at least trying to understand it. To fall in love apparently is not a thing of the body but a thing of the mind. To fall in love with God is like finding a companion that we cannot bear to live without. Many people in history fell in love with God and died for him. Is this love for God also an act of evolution?

In the books that I have researched, I found out that to fall in love is an affair that has to do with two minds, two spirits. A priest told me after my husband died that if two people love each other and one of them dies, the love still continues. My love for my husband still continues. The love for my husband can be explained because I saw him; I lived with him. How can I explain the love that I feel for God? I have never seen God. I blamed him for taking my husband away from me, but I still love him. This book is supposed to talk about a brave man, a medical doctor who was loved by so many of his patients. After his death, he let me know that he still exists. I hope that I am doing what he wants me to do by letting people know about the afterlife. To believe in the afterlife involves believing in supernatural things; it involves believing in God. When my husband was dying, he said to me, "I want to go to heaven." I am sure that he is there. My relationship with my passed husband was based on mutual love, trust, and respect.

My husband was loved by his patients because he was genuinely interested in them. He wanted to help them, and his patients knew it and did not mind coming to him from far away. Many patients came to him to talk about their personal problems. Many of my husband's patients know that I am writing this book. They encouraged me and are looking forward to reading it. I hope that the book will help them know that after this life, there is another life awaiting them. Since we know from the Bible that Jesus was always a part of the Trinity and that he was born to teach us about his Father and to open heaven for us, we should try very hard to understand his teachings and live according to them. We should also not underestimate Mary, the mother of Jesus. She also teaches us about eternity since she was taken to heaven with her body. "Mary's end attracted the greatest interest, for it promised that she had not died, that she was more than just a woman, and that she still resided in heaven alongside her Son" (Rubin 2009, 57). Some people still believe that Mary was an ordinary woman and had other children with Joseph. "The debates between emperors and priest, monks and bishops established a truth to be held by all Christians as Orthodoxy; Christ was born of a woman who was not only a virgin at His conception, but remained intact after his birth for the rest of her life" (Rubin 2009, 53).

Very important up to this day is the prophecy of Isaiah in the Old Testament. In this prophecy, it is written that the Lord himself shall give a sign, that a virgin will conceive and bear a son and shall call his name Emanuel. Traditions about Joseph, Mary's husband, appear in *The History of Joseph the Carpenter*.

> The history agrees with the gospel of James in claiming that Mary was living under Joseph's care until the moment of marriage. In his home, Mary cared for his youngest son, a sad little orphan. When she became pregnant, Joseph reacted with alarm, a moment he recalled on his deathbed: "I have never heard of a woman who had conceived without a man, or of a virgin giving birth while retaining the seal of her virginity." (Rubin 2009, 12)

The protevangelium claims that Joseph was an aged widower with children. Mark 6:3 mentions Joseph's children and Jesus this way: "This is the carpenter, surely, the son of Mary, the brother of James and Joset and Jude and Simon? His sisters too." Matthew 12:50 reads that Jesus said, "Anyone who does the will of my Father in heaven, he is my brother and sister and mother." I remember that the problem with Jesus's brothers and sisters mentioned in the Bible was once explained in church. The priest said that in those days, the stepbrothers and stepsisters would simply be called brothers and sisters. In 1 Corinthians 15:6, Paul talks about Jesus, how he appeared to five hundred of the brothers! Did Jesus have five hundred brothers? This is another example that the word *brother* was used a lot. Jesus considered brothers people that believed in God his Father in heaven. I hope that I was able to explain a little about the misconception about Mary, the mother of Jesus. I can't change whatever different religions are teaching their believers; I just wonder why there is so much misconception not only about Mary, the mother of Jesus, but also about afterlife among some Christians. If we believe in the resurrection of Christ, then we should believe in the afterlife. Paul writes in 1 Corinthians 15:14, "If there is no resurrection of the dead, Christ Himself cannot have been raised."

How can some preachers preach that after we die, we will sleep until the end of the world? Jesus told us that he would come to his Father in heaven as soon as he died. People should also learn more about Mary, the mother of Jesus. People should know that Joseph was chosen by God to look after his Son here on earth. Mary was announced to Joachim and his wife, Ann. They were supposed to become parents at a ripe old age. Theirs would be an unusual daughter that would be spoken of throughout the entire world. The Gospel of James tracks every stage of her precocious development. She has lived in the temple since the age of three until the onset of puberty. "One day…the High Priest Zachariah, guided by prayer, received a message about her future: she was to be handed over to the elderly Joseph, a widower with young children" (Rubin 2009, 10). Mary is the mother of God. She should not be reduced to an ordinary woman as some Christians are doing. I have witnessed it myself at one of the Bible study courses. Mary is helping people all over the world. Her miracles are well known. "Miracles were manifestations of

Mary's power: she bore her son miraculously, she remained a virgin miraculously even her passing from the world was a miracle" (Rubin 2009, 183). Mary's passing from the world is also teaching us about the afterlife. Miri Rubin talks about Mary's assumption to heaven in her book *Mother of God* (Rubin 2009, 56–57). I hope that Mary will receive proper recognition from people here on earth, especially from Christians.

God works in mysterious ways. When my husband found out that he was dying, his wish was that he could still be present at our daughter's wedding. Our daughter thought that she would have to call off the wedding when she found out that her father was dying. She thought that she couldn't get married if her father wouldn't walk her down the aisle. Then she got an idea: she would get married in the hospital, before her father died. The wedding was arranged in the chapel of the hospital where her father was being treated. It was very difficult to get her father dressed for the wedding and make him sit in the wheelchair as he was very weak. We finally succeeded in getting him into the chapel, and he took his daughter to the altar on the wheelchair. He also signed his name on her wedding certificate, which was his last signature in this world. My husband died just a few days later.

My husband and his daughter had their wishes fulfilled! My daughter renewed her wedding vows at another big wedding to which guests were invited previously and which was arranged a long time before my husband died. My husband was dying in the palliative care unit of the hospital, where he has been on staff since the beginning of his medical practice when the hospital first opened. It was very painful for me to think about the time when he went to the hospital to see his patients to assist in the surgeries, to deliver the babies of his patients in the middle of the night, and to go to medical meetings.

My husband always treated his patients according to the oath he took in 1965 in Prague at Charles University when he became a medical doctor. It was the words of Hippocrates, the father of scientific medicine. Hippocrates was a Greek physician born 460 BC. Hippocrates's oath is a pledge of a code of ethics taken by those about to receive a degree in medicine. It talks about the use of treatment to help the sick according to the doctor's ability and judgment but never with a view to injury or wrongdoing. The doctor promises that he will keep pure and holy both his life and his art. My husband lived his life and practiced his medicine according to those words. Some of his patients came to see him when he was dying, but they were turned back because he was too ill to see them. One family managed to get into his room when nobody was around to turn them back. My husband thanked them for coming and asked them if they brought me with them. They said that they did, that I was drinking tea in the lounge. He said, "Let her finish it." He smiled and waved them goodbye. He was too weak to talk and fell asleep. The truth was that they had not brought me with them, but they understood that he was expecting me to come. I was taking turns with my family, but it was one of the times when nobody was with him for a while.

When one of his patients and a friend of the family came to see him at the time I was with him, he told her that my husband and I were like two mules towing together without a break. She came to see her doctor and a friend for the last time. She promised to take care of our family and me in the future. It was a nice day, but it was raining in the afternoon. A beautiful, perfect rainbow stretched from one side to the other side of the big window outside my husband's hospital room. The splendid scene remained for several minutes. Our family friend is the witness to it. After my husband died, I thought about that rainbow many times. Later on, I had read in one of the books that the rainbow was a sign of God's covenant with his people. Will God send us a consolation in our grief and a promise of a happier tomorrow for my husband? Whoever does not believe that what has happened to me is a true story should calm down; it is okay. I would not believe it either if it had not happened to me, but the research that I have done should be trusted. Maybe if people would read some of the books from my research, they would believe me after all. God is the greatest mystery, and so is life after death. I would like to conclude this book with some words from Paul in 1 Corinthians 1:27–28: "It was to shame the wise that God chose what is foolish by human reckoning and to shame what is strong that he chose what is weak by human reckoning."

Jesus said:

> I am the light of the world;
> Anyone who follows me will not be walking in the dark;
> He will have the light of life. (John 8:12)

> I am the resurrection.
> If anyone believes in me, even though he dies he will live,
> And whoever lives and believes in me will never die.
> Do you believe this? (John 11:26)

> Do not let your hearts be troubled.
> Trust in God still, and trust in me. (John 14:1)

> Whoever believes in me
> Believes not in me
> But in the one who sent me,
> And whoever sees me,
> Sees the one who sent me.
> I, the light, have come into the world,
> So that whoever believes in me
> Need not stay in the dark anymore.
> If anyone hears my words and does not keep them faithfully,
> It is not I who shall condemn him,
> Since I have come not to condemn the world,

THE EPILOGUE

But to save the world:
He who rejects me and refuses my words
Has his judge already:
The word itself that I have spoken
Will be his judge on the last day.
For what I have spoken does not come from myself;
No, what I was to say, what I had to speak,
Was commanded by the Father who sent me,
And I know that his commands mean eternal life.
And therefore what the Father has told me
Is what I speak. (John 12:44–50)

Dr. Zitnansky…now laid to rest,
By far as a doctor was truly the best.
Friendly and helpful was his way,
We wish he was still with us today.
He took the time to sit with us,
And explained our results without a fuss.
He was respectful and special just one of a kind,
Never a replacement we ever shall find.
He has gone on ahead to his new Heavenly life,
While waiting the reunion of his family and wife.

Wendy L. Ross
May 24, 2012

REFERENCES

Aquinas, Thomas, and Anton C. Pegis. 1948. *Introduction to St. Thomas Aquinas.* The Modern Library.

Aquinas, St. Thomas, and Robert M. Hutchinsons. 1952. *The Summa Theologica of Saint Thomas Aquinas: Great Books of the Western World.* Encyclopedia Britannica Inc.

Behe, Michael, J. 2006. *Darwin's Black Box: The Biochemical Challenge to Evolution* (with a new afterword). New York, NY: Free Press.

Burpo, Todd and Lynn Vincent. 2010. *Heaven Is for Real: A Little Boy's Astounding Story of His Trip to Heaven and Back.* Nashville, TN: Thomas Nelson.

Chopra, Deepak, MD. 2006. *Life after Death: The Burden of Proof.* New York, NY: Harmony Books.

Clark, Mary T. 2000. *An Aquinas Reader.* New York, NY: Fordham University Press.

Collins, Francis S., Dr. *2006. The Language of God.* New York, NY: Free Press

Fenwick, Dr. Peter and Elizabeth Fenwick. 1995. *The Truth in the Light: An Investigation of Over 300 Near-Death Experiences.* London, UK: Headline Book Publishing.

Gumbel, Nicky. 2003. *Alpha: Questions of Life.* Kingsway.

Gumbel, Nicky. 1997. *The Heart of Revival.* Kingsway.

The Jerusalem Bible, Reader's Edition. 1968. Garden City, New York: Darton, Longman & Todd Ltd, Doubleday & Company Inc.

Kübler-Ross, Elisabeth, MD. 2003. *On Death and Dying*. New York: Scribner.

Kübler-Ross, Elisabeth, MD. 2008. *On Life after Death*. Berkley, ON: Celestial Arts.

Lerma, John, MD. 2007. *Into the Light*. Franklin Lakes, NJ: The Career Press.

Living Webster Dictionary. 1971. Chicago: The English language institute of America.

McBrien, Richard. 2003. *Lives of Saints*. San Francisco: Harper Collins.

Moody, Raymond A., Jr., MD. 2001. *Life after Life*. New York: NY: Harper Collins Publisher Inc.

Moody, Raymond A., Jr., MD, and Dianne Arcangel, MS. 2002. *Life after Loss*. Harper Collins Publishers Inc.

Murdoch, Dugald, John Cottingham, and Robert Stoothoff. 1985. *The Philosophical Writings of Descartes*, vol. 1 and 2. Cambridge, UK: Cambridge University Press.

Myers, Dr. F.W.H. 2001. *Human Personality and Its Survival of Bodily Death*. Charlottesville, NC: Hampton Roads Publishing Company.

Nelson, Kevin MD. 2011. *The Spiritual Doorway in the Brain: A Neurologist's Search for the God Experience*. Dutton.

Nightingale, Juliet, and Peter Fenwick, MD. 2007. Retrieved from: http://juliet.towardthelight.info/?p=475.

O'Meara, John J. 1965. *The Young Augustine*. London, UK: Longmans, Green and Co. LTD.

Osis, Karlis, PhD, and Erlendur Haraldsson, PhD. 1977. *At the Hour of Death or What They Saw…At the Hour of Death*, 3rd edition. Norwalk, MI: Hastings House Book Publishers.

Penfield, Wilder, MD, BA, MA, BSc, DSc. 1977. *No Man Alone: A Neurosurgeon's Life*. Boston, MA: Little, Brown and Company.

REFERENCES

Penfield, Wilder, OM, Litt.B, MD, FRS. 1975. *The Mystery of the Mind: A Critical study of Consciousness and the Human Brain.* Princeton, NJ: Princeton University Press.

Parnia, Sam, MD, PhD. 2006. *What Happens When We Die: A Groundbreaking Study into the Nature of Life and Death.* Carlsbad, CA: Hay House Inc.

Piper, Don, and Cecil Murphey. 2004. *90 Minutes in Heaven: A True Story of Death and Life.* Grand Rapids, MI: Revell.

Polkinghorne, John. 2007. *Quantum Physics and Theology: An Unexpected Kinship.* New Haven, CT: Yale University Press.

Rana, Fazale, PhD. 2008. *The Cell's Design: How Chemistry Reveals the Creator's Artistry.* Grand Rapids, MI: Baker Books.

Rawlings, Maurice, MD. 1978. *Beyond Death's Door.* Nashville, TN: Thomas Nelson Inc.

Ring, Kenneth PhD. 1980. *Life at Death: A Scientific Investigation of the Near-Death Experience.* Toronto, ON: Academic Press Canada Limited.

Rohr, Richard. 2009. *The Naked Now: Learning to See as the Mystics See.* New York, NY: The Crossroad Publishing Company.

Rubin, Miri. 2009. *Mother of God.* New Haven: Yale University Press.

Sabom, Michael, MD. 1998. *Light and Death: One Doctor's Fascinating Account of Near-Death Experiences.* Grand Rapids, MI: Zondervan Publishing House.

Sullivan, William F., BSc, MD, PhD. 2002. *Promise of Mercy.* Toronto, ON: University of Toronto Press.

Spong, John Shelby. 2009. *Eternal Life: A New Vision.* New York, NY: Harper Collins Publishers.

Waterfield, Robin. 2008. *Oxford World Classics: Plato—Republic; A New Translation by Robin Waterfield.* New York, NY: Oxford University Press.

Yates, Jenny. 1999. *Jung on Death and Immortality.* Princeton, NJ: Princeton University Press.

My Message to the Reader

What I want people to learn from my book is the fact that if people have a dream and the perseverance to see their dream come true, they will succeed. My husband had a dream of becoming a medical doctor since he was a child. He had no money and had to leave his parents at the age of seventeen to go to Prague, where he was accepted to study medicine, but he was happy because it was a dream come true. He had to interrupt his medical studies because he had to make money to continue. He worked as a miner for a year, which was hard work, but he did not mind. It again helped him make his dream come true. He became a medical doctor, and after a short time of being a doctor, he had to leave his country and go to Canada. He did not know any English, but after one year of taking lessons, he was able to pass his medical exams and become a medical doctor again. He was always optimistic. After he became ill, he went to his medical office everyday even if he did not feel well. He did not talk about his illness with me because he wanted me to be optimistic. Even when he saw his bad medical report, he said, "I can improve that!"

The last time he was in his office, he was there until late in the evening. He wanted to go again in the morning but collapsed and had to be taken to the hospital. He did not want to go. He said,

"I want to die at home." This was the first time he told me that he would die. During his stay in the hospital, he wanted me to pray with him. He told me that when I was with him, he was okay; but when I left him, he felt lonely. The only person my husband talked to with regard to his medical condition was one of his patients, a priest. That patient, later on after my husband died, told me that my husband was ready to die. He was not scared. I always admired my husband's exceptional will to live, even if he admitted to the priest that he was ready to die. Thinking about his optimism helped me write this book.

I wanted to write this book, especially an exceptional book where I am trying to show people that there is life after death. My husband has given me signs that he exists, and I felt that I had a responsibility to tell the public about it. It has taken me years to tell my story and show people that our loved ones still exist and that stories like mine have been documented in the past.

My husband did not let the anxiety overpower him. I am sure he felt anxious too, but he never showed it. He never said that he was afraid to die or talked about dying with me. Just before he died, I told him how much I loved him and that we would see each other again in heaven. He told me that he appreciated how much I tried to make him well during his illness. He suffered a lot, but he never complained about his pains and discomfort. His primary cancer was never found, so it was never treated. He died from his metastasis caused by the primary cancer.

My husband believed in life after death. After passing from this world, he showed me that the afterlife really exists by the signs he sent me. I am sure that he wants people to know that this life on earth is not the only one there is. I am sure that he wants people to know that they will live again after they die. It is difficult to believe it, yes, but it also is difficult to believe that we and life on earth is accidental, that everything came from nothing. It is much easier to believe that life on earth was created, was designed, because it is very complex—and our brains can't even comprehend all the details involved in the process of creation. Science can't explain everything that we want to know.

My husband was not only loved by me, he was also loved by many of his patients. When I started to write my book *Doctor's Life Beyond*, my son brought me a copy of my husband's ratings as a medical doctor. His patients were not only writing on the internet about his exceptional care during his life, they were talking about him several years after his death. My husband was called "the people's doctor." People were rating him after his death in 2007, twice in 2008, twice in 2012, and also in 2013. I am mentioning two of the comments from the ratings. In 2008, his former patient wrote,

> A great man has left us. He was a wonderful doctor, looked after our family for over thirty years. He has been interested in your whole being not just what was wrong with a certain body part. He was interested in people, he was kind, compassionate, and respectful. He was the people's doctor. He enjoyed the simple things in life, like fishing. We miss him and think of him every day, way too young to leave us.

In 2013, another former patient wrote:

> My doctor for over thirty years. He was always there, helpful and concerned. No matter what my problem, he listened and dealt with it. He listened and advised me on many matters. I wish I could have a doctor like him again. I will always remember and miss him.

More ratings can be found on the website Dr. F.P. Zitnansky G.P.—eight doctor reviews, RateMDs.com.

My husband showed me that he is still with us. My husband was also appreciated as a medical doctor in the Global Directory of Who's

Who. This distinguished edition of the registry is a leading source for recognizing the accomplishments of outstanding professional men and women in their respective fields. Recognition of this kind is shared by thousands of executive men and women throughout the United States and Canada. My husband received the application form to reserve the place with the elite local, national, and worldwide individuals who have demonstrated hard work, dedication, and perseverance in their chosen profession for several years. My husband did not want to send the application form back. He said, "I don't need it." He was a very humble man. I think that this is why his patients loved him so much.

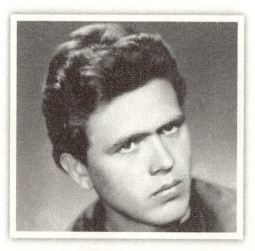

A picture of a younger Fero when he decided to work in the mines so that he could support his medical studies

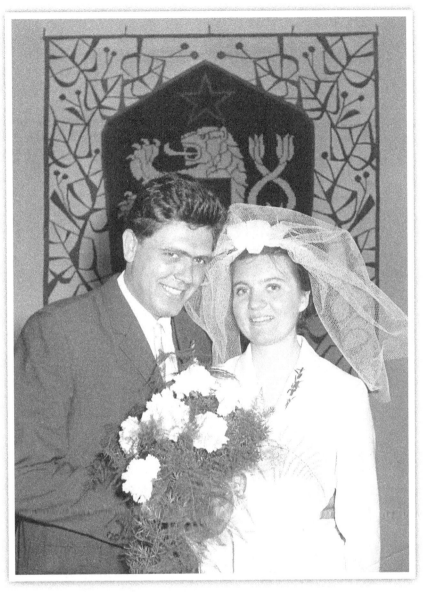

Marie and Fero's wedding picture. They forgot to go to a photographer, but luckily, a close friend was able to bring a camera and took this shot.

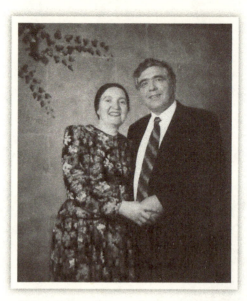

Marie and Fero in one of the medical conventions for doctors. Marie was always supportive of her husband in every situation.

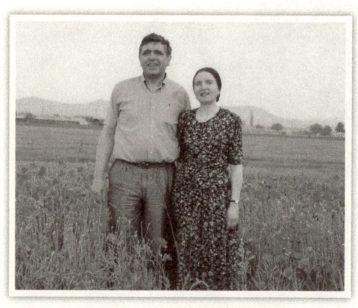

Marie's favorite picture. This was taken in Slovakia sometime in 1991. They visited the birthplace of Fero, and they saw that everything was torn down already. But to their surprise, this has now become a beautiful field with flowers, including poppy seeds.

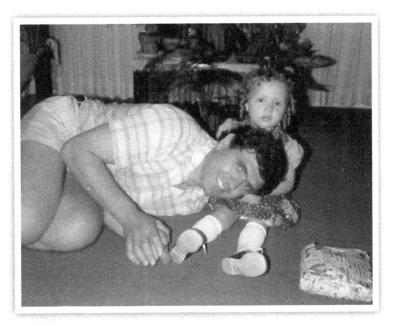

Fero always spent quality time with his children no matter what. Their daughter, Monica, was still two years old here.

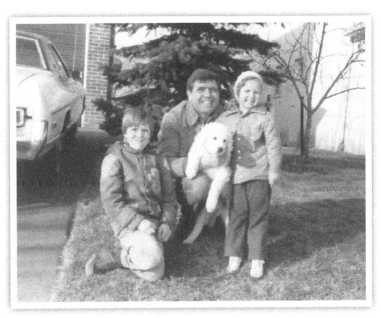

Fero with Daniel and Monica with their only dog, "Bundas," the Hungarian sheepdog

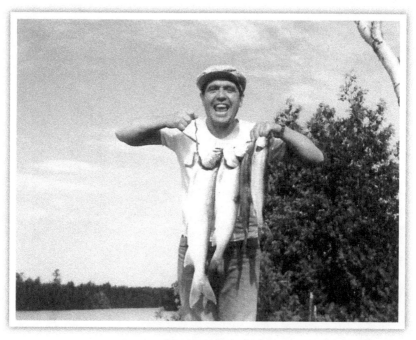

*Fero and his "other" love: fishing.
He was always happy when he went fishing.*

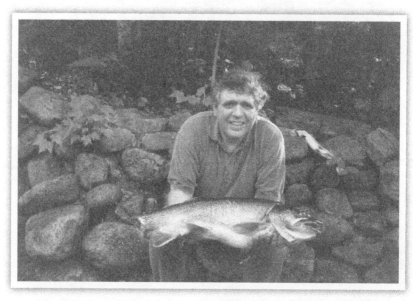

*Here, you can see Fero with his biggest catch, a lake trout,
which is now a stuffed trophy on the wall in their family cottage.*

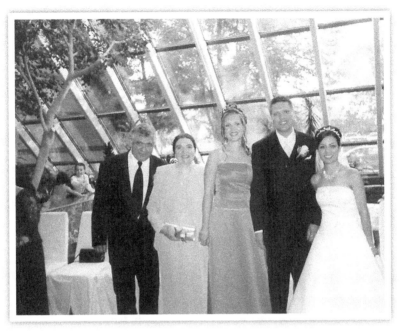

This was during Daniel's wedding, Monica in pink.

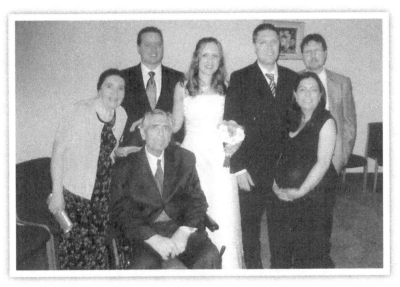

Monica's first wedding in the chapel. She wanted her father to take her to the altar; that's why they had to celebrate this wedding in the chapel, and Fero was already in wheelchair. This was also Fero's last picture together with them. He died a week after this was taken.

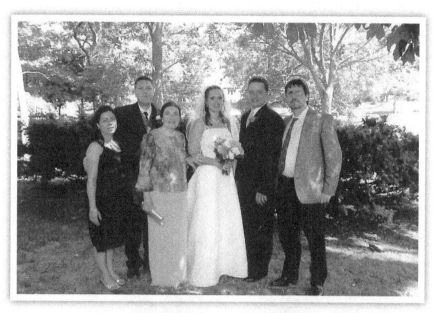

Monica's second wedding, this time in the church, but without her dad, Fero

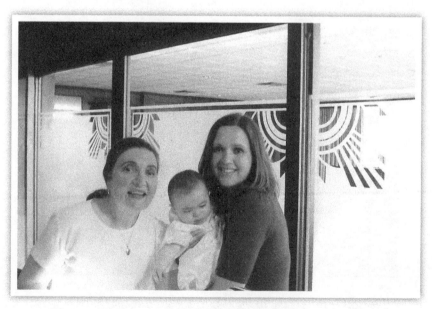

This is Marie's first grandchild, Ava, Daniel's daughter. Marie is always fascinated with how intelligent she is and truly loves her wit.

CPSIA information can be obtained
at www.ICGtesting.com
Printed in the USA
LVHW031714311019
635967LV00004B/706/P